AUTOIMMUNE DIET

THE AUTOIMMUNE MIRACLE

Discover the Secrets To Reduce Inflammation, Treat Chronic Autoimmune Disorders, Increase Metabolism, and Rebalance Your Hormones

REGINALD KELLY

Table of Contents

PART 1 7

PART 1.1: 8

The Autoimmune Problem 8

Introduction 9

Chapter 1: Origination 10

Chapter 2: Myths and Facts 13

Chapter 3: Is There a Cure? 16

Chapter 4: Histamine Intolerance 20

PART 1.2: 23

The solution 23

Chapter 5: Begin with the Gut 24

Chapter 6: Choosing the Best Foods 28

Chapter 7: Stress 31

Chapter 8: Rest 34

PART 1.3: 36

The prevention 36

Chapter 9: What to Get Rid Of 37

Chapter 10: Reduce Inflammation 41

Chapter 11: Common Mistakes 44

PART 1.4: 46

Compliment your autoimmune disease with these strategies 46

Chapter 12: Nutrition 47

Chapter 13: Exercise 52

Chapter 14: Motivation 58

Chapter 15: Food List 60

PART 1.5:	68
Meal plan and recipes	68
Chapter 16: Meal Plan	69
PART 2	84
Chapter 1: What is Inflammation Anyway?	85
Chapter 2: Inflammation causes what?	87
Chapter 3: Which Diet plan Works for you?	94
Chapter 4: Quick Recipes to try at home	98
Conclusion	104
Introduction	106
Chapter 1: Obesity and the Standard American Diet	107
The Obesity Epidemic	107
Why Are We so Fat?	109
The Problem with Calories	109
The American Diet	110
Abdominal Fat Problem: Fastest Place to Lose Weight	112
Problems and Trappings of a High-Carb Diet	112
Chapter 2: Knowledge About Proper Nutrition	113
What Causes High Blood Sugar and High Blood Pressure?	113
Lectins and Why They Are Bad	114
Chapter 3: Lack of Exercise	115
Chapter 4: Downfall of Medication	117
What Medication Does to Your Body	117
Chapter 5: Case Studies of Places with the Highest Longevity	120
Chapter 6: Who This Book Is For	122
Chapter 7: Leaky Gut Syndrome	125

Fungus Theory 125
    Intestinal Irritants 126
    Lectin Plant Proteins 126
    Whole Grains and Resistant Starches 127
Chapter 8: The Plant-Based Miracle Diet 129
    What is the Plant-Based Miracle Diet? 129
    Why Should You Get on This Diet? 132
    How to Attain a Clean Diet 133
    Scientific Mechanisms Behind the Plant-Based Diet 134
Chapter 9: Benefits of the Plant-Based Miracle Diet 136
    Stabilize Blood Sugar and Blood Pressure 136
    Other Benefits 137
Chapter 10: Other Options and Diet 138
    The Atkins Diet 138
    The South Beach Diet 138
    The Paleo Diet 139
    Why the Plant-Based Diet is Best 140
Chapter 11: Myths and Dangers 141
Chapter 12: The Importance of Nutrition 144
    Eighty Percent Diet 144
    Twenty Percent Exercise 147
Chapter 13: Safety, Side Effects, and Warnings 149
Chapter 14: The Light Dieters 152
    Changing One Meal a Day 152
Chapter 15: Intermediate Dieters 154
    Benefits, Expectations, and Results 154

Chapter 16: Hard-Core Dieters 156

Chapter 17: Going Organic 158

    Dangers of Pesticide Use and Conventional Farming 158

    GMOs 159

    Benefits of Organic Farming Techniques 161

    Benefits of Eating Organic Food 161

Chapter 18: Complement to a Healthier You 162

    The Ketogenic Diet 162

    Intermittent Fasting 163

    Exercise 166

    Accountability Partners 166

    Staying Motivated 167

    Habit Formation 168

    Foods to Focus on 169

    Foods to Avoid 170

    Supplements 171

BONUS 173

Introduction 174

Chapter One: 176

What is Plant-Based Eating? How Does It Differ From Veganism? What are The Health Benefits of Eating Plant-Based Food? 176

Chapter Two: 180

Clinical Studies: Science-Backed Proof 180

Chapter Three: 185

Basic Four-Week Meal Plan 185

Finale 197

PART 1

PART 1.1:

The Autoimmune Problem

Introduction

Many scientists and the medical community have been studying the linkage between inflammation and chronic health problems for years. Perhaps you or your loved one has recently been diagnosed with an inflammatory condition, such as Rheumatoid Arthritis or Psoriasis, and you are seeking help. Well, this is a great place to start. This book will discuss what inflammation is and some of the conditions it causes or complicates.

You may be thinking that the only solution to inflammation is the latest medication. While that may be a place to start, medication is not the whole solution. In addition to medications, there are lifestyle and dietary changes a person can do to help reduce inflammation and consequently see benefits such as reduced pain and stiffness along with some weight loss.

This book will describe several of today's anti-inflammatory diet plans. You will learn about the different types of food that have anti-inflammatory properties such as ginger and onions. Plus, there are some sample recipes included to give you a great start to an anti-inflammatory lifestyle. Finally, the suggested resources are great places to learn more about inflammation and anti-inflammatory diets.

Inflammation and inflammatory conditions are gaining more and more attention each day. Therefore, there are plenty of books on this subject on the market and we are glad you chose this one! Every effort was made to ensure it is full of as much useful information as possible. Please enjoy!

Chapter 1: Origination

An autoimmune disease is a condition that happens when the body has an unusual immune response to a healthy body part. At the moment, there are 80 known types of autoimmune diseases. Almost any part of the body can be affected by this problem. Many of the most common systems are feeling tired and having a low-grade fever. Most of the times, these symptoms will come and go.

The main cause of this problem is unknown. There are some of this disease that is hereditary, like lupus, and there are some cases where it can be triggered by an infection or environmental factor. Some of the most common autoimmune diseases are systemic lupus, rheumatoid arthritis, psoriasis, multiple sclerosis, inflammatory bowel disease, Graves' disease, type 1 diabetes, and celiac disease.

In the US, about 24 million people are affected by an autoimmune disease. Women are more often affected than men. This disease will typically start during adulthood. The first of these diseases were described during the early 1900s. A disease has to answer to Witebsky's postulates to be classified as autoimmune. This includes:

- The disease is incurable

- There is genetic evidence of clustering with other diseases

- Circumstantial clinical clues

- Evidence found in the disease reproduction in animals

- Direct evidence of disease-causing antibody or T-lymphocyte white blood cells

While doctors and scientists still seem unsure as to what causes these diseases, new research may have discovered a way to diagnose the disease better and improve treatments.

A group of scientists from Yale School of Medicine, Broad Institute of MIT and Harvard, and UC San Francisco came up with new mathematical tools to look more deeply into existing DNA. By doing so, they have found how variations, when inherited, may contribute to disease.

By using their new method to analyze data from research done on 21 different diseases, they were able to deepen the understanding of how genetics plays a role in many different disorders. They were also able to find certain immune cells that were responsible for diseases.

They looked at 39 large-scale studies known as GWAS, which means Genome-Wide Association Studies. This GWAS enlists many participants for the study to identify blocks of DNA where genetic variants may implicate a risk factor for diseases. However, this data has not really pointed to altered proteins.

Instead, they found that the DNA variation does not reside within the genes. New research has found the presence of certain genetic variants in various diseases changes gene activity patterns in a certain way that affects the function of the immune system.

They have found that there are 300 to 400 known genetic variants that work together to cause autoimmune disease, which is spread through the human genome. These genes are often located close to regions that play an important part in regulating immune function.

They now know there are two basic types of genetic diseases. One is where there is a certain mutation in a certain gene, like when it comes to muscular dystrophy, which causes the problem. But the majority of autoimmune diseases come from a complex blend of typically helpful genetic variants that everybody has, but for some, it results in illness.

Here are five main causes of autoimmune disease:

1. Hygiene theory: This country, along with others, have sanitized the environment with antibacterial soaps and many other hygiene habits that have caused a reduction in how much we are exposed

to dirt and microbes that the body is taught how to fight. This is causing an imbalance in the immune system.

2. Microbiome theory: The gut bacteria regulate how the immune system works and is being destroyed by medications and antibiotics, as well as processed foods.

3. Leaky gut syndrome: The lining of the digestive tract houses 70% of the immune system. When the cells within this lining becomes damaged, the lining may become permeable. This will cause the immune system to start reacting to medication, foods, and many other things. This means that the immune system is always ready to react.

4. Vitamin D deficiency: In some studies, this has been linked to autoimmune diseases.

5. Stress: When you have high levels of cortisol, it can affect the way the immune system works.

Chapter 2: Myths and Facts

The following will cover several myths that seem to revolve around autoimmune diseases.

Myth 1 – These disorders cannot be changed

There may be a genetic part to autoimmune disorders, but it has been discovered through epigenetics that genetic expression can be changed. For a disorder to happen, there has to be something that triggers it, but with intestinal healing and diet you can switch these genetic problems off and fix your immune system.

Myth 2 – Symptoms will not go away without medications

Many doctors will dismiss the importance of nutrition. Because of this, patients are prescribed drugs for their disorders. Instead of having to take medicines that suppress the immune system, supplements and food can support and strengthen it while healing the gut. Medications are not the only option.

Myth 3 – The side effects of medications are not important

The side effects of the drugs used for autoimmune problems are common, happen often, and are disruptive. This could mean headaches, high blood pressure, weight gain, insomnia, or any other possibility.

Myth 4 – Better gut health and digestion does not affect autoimmune disorders

The digestive system and the immune system may be two different parts of the body, but if you ignore the gut, you can cause problems. Most of the immune system is in the gut, so it is important to focus on the digestive system and heal the gut.

Myth 5 – The environment does not matter

Only 25% of your chances of developing an autoimmune disease comes from genetics. That means the other 75% is environmental. You can affect your body's response by shifting areas of your life so you can support your immune system and create a better life.

Myth 6 – Having a gluten-free diet will not change your autoimmune disorder

Going gluten-free? That is only a fad that people want to cash in on. Our ancestors have been consuming wheat for thousands of years, but all of sudden it has turned out not to be healthy for us, why?

This is what the majority of people believe when it comes to gluten and our health, and a lot of conventional practitioners do not view it any differently. If you were to mention to your doctor that you were concerned about what gluten is doing to you, and more likely than not she or he is going to say two things: "We can run a test and see if you suffer from celiac disease" and "Do you suffer from digestive problems? No? Then there's no reason for you to worry about gluten."

Thinking that gluten does not affect autoimmune conditions is probably one of the most dangerous myths that a person can have about an autoimmune disorder. Getting rid of this myth is probably of the best things that can help people with autoimmune disorders.

Myth 7 – You are doomed to have a poor quality of life if you have an autoimmune disease

"I was informed by my doctor that, over time, I would start to get weaker and weaker."

"I had to decide to tell my son he cannot bring over the grandkids because I just cannot take the risk of getting sick."

"The pain can become so bad that I have problems taking a walk with my husband."

These are some of the problems that a person who suffers from an autoimmune disease can expect to happen, sometimes frequently, but it does not mean that they are inevitable. With conventional medicine, they will end up counseling you into accepting a poor quality of life because they will make you think that your likely outcome with your condition. I'm here to let you know that this is not all inevitable.

Myth 8 – It has to do with your immune system, so there is nothing that you can do about it

Regular medical doctors will treat the autoimmune condition by helping to suppress the immune system and medicate the symptoms. If you look at The Myers Way, it will treat the autoimmune condition by helping to strengthen the immune system, which involves supporting and cleansing the gut.

Chapter 3: Is There a Cure?

A little ten-year-old girl who enjoyed riding horses went to the doctor with a severe autoimmune disease. Her joints were swollen, her skin was inflamed, her face was swollen, her immune system was hurting her whole body: her red and white blood cells, liver, blood vessels, joints, skin, muscles. She was unable to make a fist. The tip ends of her toes and fingers were cold because of Raynaud's disease that was inflaming her blood vessels. She was losing her hair, tired, and miserable. She had to take elephant dose of steroids intravenously every three weeks just so she could stay alive. She also had to take a chemo drug, methotrexate, acid blockers, aspirin, and prednisone to shut her immune system down.

Despite the medication, she did not see any results, and her tests stayed abnormal. Her regular doctors wanted to add more immune-suppressing drugs to the medication she already took. They wanted to put her on a drug that increases the risk of cancer and death from infections because it keeps the immune system from being able to fight off infections. She was not willing to accept this, so she went to get a second opinion.

Two months her first visit with the new doctor, where he figured out the underlying cause of her problems, she has quit consuming sugar, dairy, and gluten and began taking supplements, she was symptom-free. In a little less than a year, she was healthy, and her test came back normal, and she did not have to take her medications anymore.

Because of this true story, what does it mean for autoimmune disease research and how doctors approach the treatment of them? While there may be many of these diseases, they have something in common; the body starts attacking itself. So there may not be a drug that can cure these diseases, but there is obviously another way to treat them.

It used to be that medical discoveries start with a physician who has observed their patients' disease and their response to treatment. Doctors would report their findings to coworkers or would publish them as a case study. Now a lot of these case studies wind up being dismissed as a story and have ended up becoming irrelevant. People now look towards random controlled trial. The problem is this dismisses thousands of patients and doctors' experiences.

These basic discoveries can take years to be translated into regular practice. This prevents many people from accessing new therapies that they need now. The determining fact on figuring out a new approach is what the risk and benefits are to the patient.

Besides the use of antibiotics for infections and treating trauma, most medicine today tries to suppress, cover up, block, or otherwise interfere with the human body's natural workings. Doctors will not try to fix the underlying problems in the first place.

Instead, we need to ask why is the body having problems and how can it be fixed?

Functional medicine is beginning to look at things like this. This is a hidden movement that is starting to sweep the globe, and it focuses on the cause and not the symptoms. It is based in understanding the way the genes interact with the environment, and it goes past simply treating things based on labels.

For the little girl we talked about earlier, her doctors' response to her illness was to suppress the immune system, which left her open to psychiatric illness, muscle wasting, osteoporosis, infection, and cancer. But then she found somebody that asked why. He did not look at the name of the disease, but instead why the disease was there, where it started, and how to locate the cause and create a balance to her immune system.

The immune system will respond to some problem, like an allergen, toxin, or microbe, and then will go out of control. Figuring out that trigger and getting rid of it is crucial.

When the little girl's new doctor talked to her, he found that there were a lot of possible triggers. She had been exposed to Stachybotrys, a toxic mold, that was in her house. Her mother, while pregnant, had worked in limestone pits which exposed her to fluoride. She had her vaccination before 1999, which was when thimerosal was taken out of vaccines. She also took a flu shot that contains thimerosal every year. Thimerosal contains mercury, which is an immune toxin. This problem was increased by what she ate. She regularly consumed sushi and tuna, and loads of sugar, dairy, and gluten. The year before her getting sick, she had many doses of antibiotics.

The new doctor performed tests, and he found her liver function and muscle enzyme tests showed lots of damage. There were a lot of autoimmune antibodies, which means that the levels the body was attacking itself were extremely high. Markers of inflammation were also high. Her white and red blood cell count was low, as well as her vitamin D. She also has high levels of mercury; her level was 33, the normal is less than three.

After her visit to the new doctor, he placed her on an elimination diet to get rid of all the possible triggers. She got rid of gluten, sugar, and dairy. He also prescribed her a multivitamin; one that contained evening primrose oil, fish oil, folate, B12, and vitamin D. He also prescribed her Nystatin, which is a non-absorbed anti-fungal, to treat yeast. She was also given NAC (N-Acetyl Cysteine) to help her liver. The doctor also told her to stop the intravenous steroids, calcium channel blocker, and the acid blocker she had been taken.

Two months later the rash was completely gone. Her hair was growing back, and her joint pain was gone. Autoimmune markers have also improved. Her inflammation level, liver function, and muscle enzymes were normal again.

At her next visit, she was given probiotics to help her digestive function and gut health. He also gave her DMSA (Dimercaptosuccinic Acid) to remove the mercury from her cells and tissues. She was also given herbs to help her adrenal gland and so that she could stop taking prednisone.

After seven months, all of her test were perfect, including her white blood cells count. Mercury levels had decreased from 33 to 16. By month 11, her mercury levels were at 11. She did not have to take any of her medications and was feeling normal, happy, and could ride a horse again.

Some people may be able to dismiss this as a spontaneous remission, or claim that the testing was unconventional, or the treatment unproven. But there is a shimmer of hope that this could work, and it can help to recover from a devastating and debilitating disease.

This little girl's story is not one in a million. This approach of figuring out and getting rid of triggers for a disease like hidden allergens, toxins, or microbes, and supporting how the body functions with herbs and nutrients and "pro" drugs are more than just an idea that has to be proven. This is a movement that thousands of practitioners are using. It is an approach that has already helped thousands of patients around the world. Doctors have the knowledge and the methods, so why not apply them?

Chapter 4: Histamine Intolerance

Do you ever have unexplained anxiety or headaches? Do you have irregular menstrual cycles? When you drink red wine, does your face flush? Do you experience a runny nose or itchy tongue when you eat eggplants, bananas, or avocados? If you said yes to any one of these questions, then you may have histamine intolerance.

Histamine is a chemical that works with the immune system, central nervous system, and digestion. It is a neurotransmitter that communicates messages from the body up to the brain. It also works with stomach acid, which breaks down the food in the stomach.

You are probably most familiar with what histamine is as it relates to the immune system. If you have seasonal allergies or a food allergy, you probably know that antihistamine drugs such as Benadryl, Zyrtec, or Allegra will give you fast relief. The reason for this is because histamine's job within the body is to create an immediate inflammatory response. It's a red flag for the immune system and tells your body that there is a potential risk.

Histamine will swell or dilate the blood vessels so that the white blood cells can get to problems and fix it. The buildup of histamine is what causes you to have a headache, and leaves you feeling miserable, flushed, and itchy. This is a natural immune response, but if your body does not break down histamine correctly, you may end up developing histamine intolerance.

Since histamine travels through the blood, it can affect your cardiovascular system, brain, skin, lungs, and gut causing many different problems making it hard to diagnose.

Symptoms of histamine intolerance can include:

- Tissue swelling

- Fatigue
- Hives
- Abnormal menstrual cycle
- Difficulty breathing, nasal congestion, sneezing
- Flushing
- Abdominal cramps
  - Vomiting, nausea
  - Anxiety
  - Difficulty regulating body temp
  - Accelerated heart rate or arrhythmia
  - Dizziness or vertigo
  - Hypertension
  - Easily awoken, difficulty falling asleep
  - Migraines or headaches

Things that can cause high levels of histamine mean are histamine-rich foods, diamine oxidase deficiency, fermented alcohol, GI bleeding leaky gut, bacterial overgrowth, and allergies.

Besides the histamine that the body naturally produces, some foods contain histamine or block the enzyme that helps to break histamine down.

Once histamine has been formed, it will either be stored or broken down by a certain enzyme. In the central nervous system, histamine is broken down typically by histamine N-methyltransferase, while in the digestive tracts it will be broken down by diamine oxidase. Even though both enzymes work to break down histamine, it has been found that DAO (Diamine Oxidase) is the main enzyme that works to breaks down ingested histamine. If you have a deficiency in DAO, you will probably suffer from histamine intolerance.

You can get tested for histamine intolerance to make sure if you suffer from it. The first you can do on your own: elimination and reintroduction. Start by removing foods high in histamine for 30 days and start reintroducing them one at a time. You can get a blood test that will test your histamine and DAO levels. If you have a high ratio of histamine to DAO, then you may be ingesting a lot of histamines, and your DAO is too low to break it down.

If you can get a blood test, you can start eating a diet that is low in histamine and start taking a DAO supplement with each meal. If you notice that your symptoms go away, then you may have low DAO.

To treat histamine intolerance, get rid of foods high in histamine from one to three months. Start taking a DAO supplement, which you will take two pills at every meal. However, remember, consult your doctor before taking any supplement. The most important thing is to figure out the cause of your histamine intolerance. If you take a medication that is causing this intolerance, talk with your doctor to see about getting you off these medications. The most common cause is gluten intolerance and SIBO, which will cause leaky gut. If that is your problem, then you can heal your gut, and you will not have to eliminate foods, and you will not have to take DAO.

If you find that you do suffer from histamine intolerance, the good news is that you may not have to stay away from histamine foods for forever. This is just a short-term fix until DAO or histamine levels get back to normal. Depending on you, you could find that you can handle some foods better than others, so make sure you stay optimistic.

PART 1.2:

The solution

Chapter 5: Begin with the Gut

While it is easy to overlook the health of the gastrointestinal system (GI), it still contains ten times more healthy bacteria than any other part of the body. It helps to promote elimination and healthy digestion, supports metabolism, and protects us from infection.

Unfortunately, most people had inadequate beneficial bacteria and took many damaging bacteria, and they lack diversity. This is mainly due to a bad diet, but may be caused from:

- Current body and health composition – poor disease status

- Inadequate bacterial acquisition at birth – C-section, parent gut health, mother's diet during pregnancy, transition from breast milk to solid food

- Environment toxins – BPA, arsenic, herbicides, PCBs, pesticides

- Chronic stress

- Over-medicating – antacids, antidepressants, NSAIDs, birth control, antibiotics

All of this will lead to unbalanced gut flora, and this increases the chance of permeability. This is because the same things that hurt out gut flora and compromise the gut barrier; while infections and bad bacteria can prosper can do the same.

The bad part about it is that for some of the problems, it is presented as something that seems harmless such as excess gas, IBS (Irritable Bowel Syndrome), heartburn, and bloating, but for others, it can mean some serious things like chronic inflammation of the nervous or brain system, bowl, joints, or skin.

This is caused by the fact that even though the gut is inside the body, it is really an external organ that's role is to keep harmful substances out of the body. So if the barrier is becoming compromised, foreign molecules can pass into the bloodstream, and problems can start. The body will then launch into an immune response for protection, but ends up hurting your tissues and organs. Recent research has found that leaky gut is connected to hundreds of medical conditions including:

- Chronic kidney disease
- Dermatitis
- Schizophrenia
- Parkinson's
- Allergies and asthma
- Type 1 diabetes
- Chronic fatigue
- Lupus
- Multiple sclerosis
- Social anxiety and depression
- IBD
- Autism, ADHA, and Tourette's
- Rheumatoid arthritis
- Fibromyalgia

This tends to be where some will get upset and quit listening. This because if it is true, which research suggest it is, the underlying problem to your health was caused by you, since your upset gut was caused by what you did; whether exposing yourself to bad things, eating certain foods, or over medicating.

But the thing is, it is not actually your fault.

The only thing you are guilty of is listening to "experts" and choosing the best choices you were given. These are the same options that everybody else was faced with. Unfortunately for you, or your relatives, may not have as much genetic protection as others. Or you just did not start out with a strong shot from the get-go.

This should give you hope. It means that you can change your performance and health. If you are dealing with or taking care of someone who is dealing with a gastrointestinal problem, mental disorder, or neurological condition, you can potentially change your life.

A little honesty here though, there is no guarantee that it will help, but the evidence makes us believe that this kind of problems does start in the gut. Helping the gut out can give you improvements.

While not every disease may be because of leaky gut, and not everybody has leaky gut, but evidence shows us that an old hypothesis is not quackery. So there is really no reason why you shouldn't be doing something to promote gut health and improve the integrity of the gut lining.

To help heal your gut, you can follow this four-part system known as the 4 R's:

Remove

Get rid of all the bad. The goal here is to remove the things that negatively affect your gut like drugs, caffeine, alcohol, infections, and inflammatory foods.

Inflammatory foods can include sugar, eggs, soy, corn, dairy, and gluten because they can lead to sensitivities. An elimination diet is a good starting point to figure out the foods that cause you the most problems. This is where you remove foods for a couple of weeks and then start to add them back in and to notice how your body responds.

Infections may be caused by bacteria, yeast, or parasites. It's important to get a comprehensive stool analysis to determine your levels of good bacteria and possible infections that you could have. Getting rid of the infections may mean treatments with antifungal supplements, antifungal medication, anti-parasite medication, herbs, and antibiotics, if completely necessary.

Replace

Add in good. Start adding in the things that are important for proper absorption and digestion that may have become depleted by aging, diseases, drugs, or diet. This could include bile acids, hydrochloric acid, and digestive enzymes that are needed for proper digestion.

Reinoculate

Restoring the good bacteria to reestablish a good balance of beneficial bacteria is important. This can be done by taking a probiotic that contains good bacteria like lactobacillus and bifidobacteria species. 25 to 100 billion units each day is a good range to go for. A prebiotic supplement or eating foods that are high in soluble fiber is also important.

Repair

Give your system the nutrients that it needs to help fix the gut itself. A great supplement for that is L-glutamine, which is an amino acid that helps the gut wall lining. Other types of nutrients are vitamin E, A, and C, Omega-3 fish oils, and zinc, along with herbs like aloe vera and slippery elm.

No matter the problems you are facing, the 4 R's can help to heal up your gut. Lots of inflammatory and chronic illnesses respond positively to this in just a short amount of time.

Chapter 6: Choosing the Best Foods

Most autoimmune diseases are often treated with immunosuppressive medications, which will only cause bigger risks for the body. The good thing is, more research has found that a dietary change can lower the symptom severity, stop disease progression, and may even keep the problem from ever starting.

Omega-3 fats can reduce inflammation. Average Americans today will have a diet that has an unbalanced proportion of omega-6 and omega-3 fatty acid. Ideally, the body needs more omega-3 fatty acids because they provide an anti-inflammatory effect. Omega-6 fatty acids are important if they are in higher concentrations in the diet from processed foods, and with large amounts of vegetable oils, it can cause an increase in molecules which can cause inflammation.

Some individuals that suffer from various autoimmune diseases have seen an improvement in their symptoms by taking a fish oil supplement. People that have rheumatoid arthritis had a 73% decrease in drug treatment. Patients that had Crohn's disease had a 60% decrease in their relapse rate.

Fatty acids help to decrease an immune system that caused inflammation. Fatty acids can suppress the antibodies that cause an immune system alarm for defense and helps to improve pathways of the cells that cause inflammation.

If you tend to experience symptom flare-ups without any reason, oxalates may cause inflammation. If you can detect that oxalates are causing your autoimmune response, then you can heal yourself quicker.

Oxalates are compounds that naturally occur in nature that is found in protein alternatives like some veggies and fruits, nuts, grains, and soy. Some of these foods can be added to a healthy diet, if you have an unhealthy gut you can experience oxidative stress, nutrient deficiency, and chronic inflammation that can damage the body.

Antioxidants can help reduce inflammation. If there is an increase in antioxidants, it can decrease oxidative stress, which causes tissue damage, and that means it is directly correlated with the reduction of inflammation, autoimmune disease, and chronic illness. A study discovered that a diet that was supplemented with antioxidants and was lower in caloric and fat intake delayed the start of Lupus symptoms by stimulating the immune system.

Antioxidants will help the brain from oxidative stress which is known to cause loss of cognitive function and aging. Maintaining a healthy mind and gut interaction is important for healthy vitality and aging.

Vitamins that provide antioxidants have anti-inflammatory properties that inhibit cytokine activity for diseases that are autoimmune, which are what signals an inflammatory response in cells. Herbs that have high levels of antioxidants, like curcumin which comes from turmeric, have shown to have the same anti-inflammatory response as synthetic drugs like aspirin.

B-12, folate, and B-6 all have antioxidant properties. Vitamin B-6 has been found to inhibit macrophages from taking over foreign matters that are associated with autoimmune problems. A deficiency in B-6 has been shown to correlate with increased sensitivity to oxalates contained in food.

A person with the MTHFR gene (Methylenetetrahydrofolate reductase) mutation has a lower ability to produce important antioxidant glutathione. This is crucial for immune modulation and detoxification. This makes them at a higher risk of developing chronic inflammatory diseases and autoimmune problems.

Stay away from nightshades. This includes any pepper, white potato, and tomatoes and they help an unhealthy autoimmune response. Nightshades will increase calcium deposits within tissues which can cause chronic inflammation which will cause more problems and health consequences.

Damage to the liver and kidneys can cause autoimmune diseases like diabetes and rheumatoid arthritis. Not all people have a negative response to nightshades. However, people that have autoimmune problems will struggle with the foods.

Here are some nutritional tips:

- Drink purified water
- Buy organic. Toxins found in pesticides can destroy gut health
- Avoid foods that do not come from nature
- Switch vegetable oils to cold pressed oils like coconut and olive
  - Eliminate refined sugars
  - Commit to prebiotic and probiotic supplements
  - Get rid of coffee and switch to organic teas

Let's touch on that last point, coffee. Coffee tends to negatively affect people with an autoimmune disorder. Coffee comes from a seed and is not recommended when it comes to an autoimmune diet. Seeds and nuts typically cause the least problems, so you may be able to add them back in.

For somebody with gluten intolerance or celiac disease, coffee can be harmful to them. Coffee is a cross-reactive food to gluten, which means that some bodies will view coffee the same as gluten.

Coffee will also overstimulate the adrenal glands which cause an increase in adrenal fatigue. People will get into the habit of use caffeine as their energy source, which gives short-term benefits but long-term problems. Decaf is not really any better than caffeinated because of the chemicals that are used to get rid of the caffeine.

Some good alternatives to coffee are rooibos tea, herbal teas, ginger infusion, and bone broth.

Chapter 7: Stress

Stress has a strong connection with many health problems such as autoimmune problems, insomnia, heart disease, diabetes, and obesity. Internal inflammation also plays a role in the release of stress hormones, adding to an imbalance. If stress levels are not fixed, then serious problems can happen over time. When you experience a fight or flight response, cortisol is released. Whenever we experience danger, no matter how insignificant, the body will go into survival mode. The body will signal the adrenal cortex to release cortisol. While we can feel the increase in adrenaline, your body will also experience:

- Increase in glucose production
- Certain cells will not respond to insulin
- Production of insulin is reduced
- Tissue growth and repair is stopped
  - Arteries narrow causing an increase in blood pressure

Mental stress leads to an increase of cortisol which can cause a chronic anti-inflammatory response. This can lead to the degradation of the digestive tract wall which can cause inflammation causing more cortisol to be released. This means that stress is only going to cause more problems, especially if you suffer from an autoimmune disease.

Stress and anxiety are like a monster under the bed that steals a peaceful night's sleep of almost 70 million Americans. Things like anxiety sabotage confidence and turn the stomach into knots and hurt your overall well-being. Here are five tips to help you get your stress and anxiety under control.

1. Remind yourself that it will pass

Your boss wants a report from yesterday's work, the baby is sick, and the laundry is piling up. Does any of this sound familiar? Nobody that is taking care of their own life is going to be completely stress-free, and too much is going to lead to difficulty breathing, upset stomach, dread, nervousness, and excessive worry. The first step to overcoming these feelings is to understand that you are going through something common and what is known as anxiety. Even though the negative emotion is uncomfortable, these feelings are going to pass. If you fight these feelings, it will cause worse emotions. If you accept them, you will notice that you start feeling better.

2. Start Self-Soothing

Imagine yourself walking through the woods, and you end up meeting a bear, or worse, your boss demanding a report. When faced with a situation like this, the body's sympathetic nervous system will trigger physiological changes. The breath quickens, adrenaline is released, and the heart starts to race. This is supposed to help us escape life-threatening emergency. Except when the threat is only imagined, it causes an unnecessary response. You can use diaphragmatic breathing for relaxation. You cannot manually reduce your heart rate; you can use deep breathing techniques to lower your pulse rate.

Positive self-talk is another way to self-soothe. Instead of using the comments that you normally say to yourself like "that was a stupid mistake," try using positive phrases. Try using, "I'm safe now," "I can make it through this," and other positive sayings.

Muscle relaxation is another great option. To do this, go through your body and tight and then release your muscles. This will help the stress to release from the muscles, helping you to relax.

3. Check your diet

The things that you consume plays a big part in your emotional state. Alcohol and caffeine-containing foods exacerbate anxiety and stress more than any other. Do not abruptly eliminate them though. This can cause withdrawal symptoms, which can cause more problems. It's best if you slowly reduce them.

4. Get moving

Most everybody understands that exercise is important for good health. Over the past few decades, research has found that exercise can be more effective than any medication. Keeping a healthy, non-obsessive, regular exercise routine can help to increase energy levels, enhance self-esteem, improve mood, and reduce stress. When you are exercising, the body will release a chemical called endorphins which interact with brain receptors causing euphoric feelings and will lower physical pain.

5. Sleep more

Pretty much everybody will feel crabby when he or she do not get a good night's sleep. Bad sleep is a very common emotional problem, and it's hard to figure out which one came first: poor sleep or stress. One study has shown that losing only a few hours of sleep can cause an increase in exhaustion, sadness, anger, and stress.

Chapter 8: Rest

We touched on sleep in the last chapter, now let's look at why it is so important. A person cannot be completely healthy if they do not get enough sleep. As we are sleeping, the body repairs and maintains itself, which is important in maintaining health. Sleep keeps the organs working, improves immunity, gives us energy, boosts mood, helps with stress, and enhances mental clarity.

Sleep deprivation can have these effects on the body:

- Increased risk of death
- Systemic inflammation
- Mental and mood problems
- Cognitive decline
- Obesity and weight gain
- Impaired immunity

Even though we understand the importance of sleep, our culture is still willing to sacrifice sleep for productivity. Most everybody will force his or her body to stay up past sundown, which is the time when the body expects to go to bed. Along with devices like phones and computers, this all can mess up our balance of hormones that you need to maintain and induce sleep. Most people will miss the ideal time to go to sleep, get a second wind, which will cause problems falling asleep. Another problem in our culture is that we do not let our self get enough sleep. Most people get around six hours of sleep when we really need eight to nine. This causes you to wake up feeling unrefreshed and exhausted and need of coffee.

Getting a good night sleep seems to be difficult for the average person, so imagine the difficulty for a person with an autoimmune disease. The stress, pain, and depression that is associated with autoimmunity can make getting a full and good night sleep difficult. The body has more inflammation and repair that it is faced with every day, meaning that sleep is even more important to those with an autoimmune disease than an average person. Because it's so important, getting adequate rest should be an important part of managing your autoimmune disease.

Here are some tips that will help you to get a better night's sleep:

- Make use of stress-management tools throughout your day

- Reduce the amount of exposure you have to blue light right before you go to bed. Make sure that you turn off all screens a few hours before you go to bed.

- Think about making your bedroom a technology-free zone. You may find it easier to sleep if you do not take your devices to bed with yours.

- Stay away from stimulants like sugar and caffeine before bed.

- Make your sleeping environment dark and comfortable. If you cannot get your room completely dark, you may want to get an eye mask or blackout curtains.

- Come up with a bedtime ritual. This could be anything. You could take a little walk after dinner, take a bath, and read a book before going to bed. Find a relaxing routine that you do every day so that your body can calm down and you will be able to slip off to sleep.

- Do not go to sleep with a full belly. Make sure you have a few hours after your last meal before you try to go to sleep. This will give you system adequate digestion time.

PART 1.3:

The prevention

Chapter 9: What to Get Rid Of

We have looked at many of the reasons for autoimmune diseases, and I have given you some ways to reverse symptoms associated with these diseases and to balance the immune system.

Now let's look at the top triggers that can create flare-ups that will cause devastating symptoms. The following foods probably need to be removed from your diet. This goes for somebody with a full-blown disease like Hashimoto's, celiac, or Crohn's disease, or a common "autoimmune spectrum disorder" such as IBS or acne. You need to be aware of the possible landmines that can cause an inflammatory response.

1. Gluten

This "G" word is one of the proteins found in rye, spelt, barley, wheat, and many other grains. This protein has been linked to many different risks for autoimmunity.

There are a lot of doctors and people that believe you have to have celiac disease to be intolerant to gluten. When the lab results tell them they do not have celiac, the doctors tell them they do not need to cut out gluten. This kind of misinformation is what keeps people struggling with their autoimmune conditions.

For a lot of people that suffer from autoimmune problems, it does not take a piece of pasta or bread to cause problems. Food that was cross-contaminated with gluten can cause problems for them.

2. Gluten-free grains

Most people that have autoimmune problems will have already cut out gluten, but they will still consume rice, oats, and corn. As well-intentioned as this may be, this kind of grains is still just as damaging as gluten can be, and maybe even more so.

The proteins found in these ground are a lot like gluten, which is just like play Russian roulette for a person that suffers from an autoimmune condition. Similar to having a gluten sensitivity, these symptoms do not have to be gastrointestinal. Any sort of autoimmune symptom flare-up can happen when these grains are consumed.

Everybody is different, so it could be helpful that you run immunological blood tests to see the things that your body cross-reacts with.

3. Quinoa

One of the favorites within the health community is the pseudo-grain quinoa. They contain high levels of the protein saponin which can cause problems for the lining of the gut, which causes an immune response within the body. If you soak and rinse the quinoa, it can reduce its damaging effects to the gut, but for people with autoimmune conditions, it may not be enough.

4. Toxins

The environment is full of toxins that 100 years ago were unknown. Studies have found that these toxins play a part in autoimmune problems like autoimmune thyroiditis.

5. Sugar

It probably does not come as a surprise that sugar would be on this list, but this does not just include the stereotypical junk food. There are lots of "healthy" junk foods out there that are popular within the health community that can cause negative effects to autoimmune problems.

Healthier sounding foods like agave nectar and organic turbinado sugar written on a food label may make it sound natural and earthy, but to your immune system sugar is still sugar.

6. Chocolate

This very yummy food can create a lot of damage to people that live with an autoimmune condition. Research has found that people who suffer from an autoimmune disease may be affected negatively by the consumption of chocolate.

7. Dairy

Casein is one of the main proteins that are found in milk, and many other dairy products may cause a trigger for inflammation within the body. Getting rid of the dairy proteins within clarified butter or ghee can give some people a safer alternative. Some autoimmune disorders can handle fermented dairies, such as kefir or grass-fed whole yogurt.

8. Nightshades

This plant group contains spices, goji berries, eggplants, potatoes, peppers, and tomatoes that contain alkaloids within their skin. These can cause the body to have an inflammatory response.

9. SIBO

SIBO stands for *small intestinal bacterial overgrowth*. This occurs when the normal bacteria that live in the large intestines start to travel to the small intestines. This can end up leading to many localized autoimmune spectrum conditions like acid reflux and IBS. Chronic SIBO may also lead to leaky gut, which will cause more autoimmune problems through the entire body.

10. Weakened microbiome

Most of your immune system lives within what is called the microbiome. This is a highly sophisticated gut ecosystem that is made up of bacterial colonies. This microbiome is what controls, not only the immune system, but also the genetic expression, brain, and hormones.

Fungal, parasitic, and yeast infections can a be implicated in many autoimmune problems like MS and Parkinson's. It is important that you understand these symptoms do not have to show up as gastrointestinal.

11. Leaky gut syndrome

Functional medicine believes that an increase in the permeability of the gut lining is a precursor to developing autoimmunity. Everything else that I have mentioned can lead to a leaky gut. This means that leaky gut is also seen as a casual trigger, but the effect of this will proceed from an autoimmune condition.

When the gut is damaged, any undigested food proteins, as well as bacterial endotoxins, will be able to pass through the protective lining of the gut, which will cause an autoimmune reaction throughout the entire body.

Basically, you need to find what is your underlying personal trigger. This can help eliminate years of unnecessary suffering that a lot of autoimmune suffers have to go through. I cannot stress this enough; everybody is different, so you need to find what works before for your unique case.

Chapter 10: Reduce Inflammation

Chronic inflammation plays a huge role in many diseases, like Crohn's disease, autoimmune diseases, type-2 diabetes, as well as the three top killers: stroke, cancer, and heart disease. Research is looking into the line between brain disorders like dementia and Alzheimer's disease and inflammation. Diet, lifestyle change, and exercise are powerful tools to fight inflammation. Here are some ways you can get rid of inflammation.

Balance Omega Fats

People eat too many inflammations-causing omega-6 fats that are found in fast food, processed foods, vegetable oils like corn and sunflower and not eating enough inflammation-soothing omega-3 fats like olive oil, canola, walnuts, flaxseeds, tuna, and salmon. A diet high in omega-6s and low in omega-3s will increase inflammation in the body. To balance your omega fats, choose fresh, unprocessed food. Swap the sunflower or corn oil for canola or olive oil and load your plate with foods that are rich in omega-3s. If you eat one source of Omega-3s each day, you will be doing great things for inflammation. Omega-3s boost some proteins that slow down inflammation and reduce the number of proteins that cause inflammation. If you just cannot get four grams with food, ask about a supplement. Taking a fish-oil supplement each day will reduce inflammatory markers by about 14 percent.

Yoga

People who practiced 75 to 90 minutes of yoga twice a week have lower levels of interleukin-6 and C-reactive protein (CRP). These are two inflammatory markers. Practicing yoga can reduce stress responses. Researchers think yoga benefits people because it minimizes stress-related changes.

Eat More Soy

Eating 25 grams of soy each day can reduce the risk of inflammation-driven cardiovascular disease. There can be results with consuming just half that amount. Lunasin, a peptide found in tofu and soymilk when combined with other soy protein, can quell inflammation. If you have hormone-sensitive conditions like endometriosis and breast cancer, ask your doctor before increasing your soy intake.

Get a Massage

A massage is more than a treat. It is all a part of being healthy. Getting a 45-minute massage can lower two key inflammation-promoting hormones. Massages can decrease inflammatory substances by increasing how much disease-fighting white blood cells. It can lower stress hormones. These results are seen after just one massage.

Limit Bad Fats

Trans-fatty acids are linked to an increase in body inflammation. Trans fats are found in foods like margarine, crackers, cookies, and fried foods. If the label says zero-gram trans-fat, it might still have about one-half gram per serving. If you eat more than one serving, you are eating several grams. Look for partially hydrogenated oil on the label. If you see this, it has trans fats. Cut back on saturated fats, too. Replace butter with olive oil and be choosy about proteins. Eat more lean proteins like plant-based proteins such as beans, white-meat poultry, and fish.

Eat Greens

Here is another reason to eat your greens, nuts, and whole grains: these foods are all rich in magnesium. Have your doctor check your magnesium level with a blood test. Most people who have high inflammation markers have low magnesium levels. People who have conditions that are associated with inflammation, like diabetes and heart disease have low magnesium levels. Eating magnesium-rich foods will help to lower inflammation.

Get Rid of Stress

If you are easily frazzled, you are opening the door for inflammation. A study found that people who have strong emotional reactions to stress will have a greater increase in circulating interleukin-6 when stressed. Stress will increase the heart rate and blood pressure, and this makes your blood vessels work harder. You are pounding on them and causing damage. If too much damage happens, inflammation persists.

Get More Sleep

If you do not get a minimum of six hours of restful sleep every night, you are susceptible to inflammation. Getting less than six hours of sleep has been linked to increased levels of three key markers like fibrinogen, CRP, and interleukin-6.

Exercise

Eating right and losing some weight with exercise is a great way to lower your inflammation. Working out can lower inflammation even if you do not lose any weight. Why? Exercising at 60 to 80 percent of your heart rate can lower the level of CRP which is a key inflammation marker. Think about taking a brisk walk where you can talk but not hold a full conversation.

Drink Green Tea

If coffee is your go-to beverage, you may not want to get rid of tea, especially green tea. Green tea is full of antioxidants that help to slow down inflammation. Researchers found that green tea can stop the oxidative stress and inflammation that results from it. People who drank 500 mg of green tea daily halved their stress levels.

Chapter 11: Common Mistakes

Many people who have autoimmune disease manage their condition with exercise and diet. They stay away from foods that cause inflammation, take their medicines, and use natural remedies. Many people struggle with their illness daily. Here are some things that can make your disease worse without you even realizing it.

Eating Specific Foods

Most people's first thought is to eat organic and cleaner foods. Just because the food is labeled as organic does not mean you need to eat it.

Nightshades like peppers, potatoes, and tomatoes can cause inflammation in people with an autoimmune disorder. Grains, dairy, and eggs can cause inflammation as well. These are hard to digest, and this causes flare-ups to your condition.

No Live Probiotics

People who have an autoimmune disease have imbalances of gut flora. This leads to a digestive condition like Candida. Be sure that fermented vegetables are part of your diet. Sauerkraut and kimchi are great sources of good bacteria as well as non-dairy kefirs and apple cider vinegar.

Heavy Metal Toxicity

This is common in soda cans, smoke, paint, personal hygiene products, and seafood. These are hard to stay away from.

Heavy metals are associated with different health conditions like autoimmune diseases. Heavy metal toxicity causes many symptoms like fatigue, paralysis, memory problems, chronic pain and other conditions.

Be sure you get tested for heavy metal toxicity if you have an autoimmune disorder. Getting rid of these metals could make a huge difference in your life.

No Live Enzymes

The body makes many different digestive enzymes but digesting foods can deplete your enzyme stores. Many diets do not replenish their depleted enzymes. Smoothies, fresh juices, and salads are a great place to begin promoting digestive health.

Other factors might contribute to making autoimmune conditions worse like prescription medicines, vitamin D deficiency, etc.

Fixing these issues might be the key to better health, even if they do not make your disease go away totally.

PART 1.4:

Compliment your autoimmune disease with these strategies

Chapter 12: Nutrition

Some common questions about Autoimmune Protocol are: should it be done alone or should it be layered with other diets like a low carb, Candida, SCD, GAPS, or low-FODMAP diets? This chapter will discuss the different diets. You should always consult your doctor before changing or adding anything to what your doctor has told you to do.

Low-Carb Diet

The low-carb diet has different versions, but the main distinction is if the number of carbs is enough to put a person into ketosis. This is when the body relies on ketones and glucose to supply energy to the body. It is achieved by eating less than 25 grams of carbs each day. This is a relative number as some can produce ketosis by eating a higher number of carbs, others have to eat less. Many consider a diet that is between 50 and 100 grams of carbs each day a low-carb diet. Some say a low-carb diet is effective against neurological disorders and some cancers. Others have success with weight loss or regaining insulin sensitivity by eating a low-carb diet.

The Candida and SCD Diet

These diets have different protocols but share a pathogen-specific approach. Their purpose is to get rid of foods that feed the overgrowth in the gut like starches even those that are included in the autoimmune protocol such as tapioca, squash, and sweet potatoes, grains, milk, fruit juice, sweeteners, fruit, and other foods.

These can help eliminate symptoms for people who have overgrowths but neither can eliminate pathogens by themselves. If someone experiences these symptoms when eating certain foods, do not blindly go one of the different pathogen-specific diets. Test the diet, do not guess. Many who can help successful recover from overgrowths know which pathogen they are fighting. Some might need to be approached from different angles like probiotics, antifungals, herbal or prescription antibiotics. Work with someone who is experienced in this area.

These diets do not eliminate many allergens, and that is a problem for some who have autoimmunity like nightshades, dairy, and eggs.

GAPS Diet

This is similar to the Candida and SCD diet since it incorporates a specific pathogen approach, but it does pinpoint allergens and gut-healing nutrients. This diet contains well-cooked meat, broth, and vegetables for a certain amount of time until more foods are added one at a time to determine if they can be tolerated. The first ones to be introduced are nuts, ghee, fermented dairy, egg yolks, probiotics, and fermented vegetables. This diet is used with neurological conditions and autism and has been used with different chronic health problems.

Low-FODMAP Diet

This diet gets rid of short-chain fermentable carbs that feed the overgrowth of bacteria in the gut. Many problems like cramps, gas, bloating, diarrhea, constipation, and IBS use this diet to get their digestive issues under control. All high-FODMAP foods are gotten rid of for several weeks and then reintroduced slowly to see how well the body will tolerate it.

The low-FODMAP has been used for people with Candida, SIBO, malabsorption, and other imbalances. It helps with symptoms of digestive overgrowth, it is not an autoimmune specific diet and includes some allergens like nightshades, nuts, and eggs. For people who suffer from these issues and cannot get them relieved by AIP (Autoimmune Protocol), adding a low-FODMAP for a couple of weeks could be helpful.

Low-FODMAP is effective when managing an overgrowth, is not effective by itself to treat an overgrowth. It needs to be layered with an AIP to be effective.

There is a lot of information about AIP, but other's journeys are not your journey. Take it one step at a time. Remember in time you will find out things about your health that will allow you to make progress but it might not happen suddenly.

It is advisable for people who have an autoimmune disorder to supplement with minerals and vitamins.

Vitamin D

The best source of vitamin D is sunshine. It can be supplemented by other means. The immune system is impacted by vitamin D within your system.

This vitamin gets converted into a hormone known as calcitriol. This will turn on an antibacterial protein and a defense against any unrecognized invaders.

It is important to prevent an overreaction to these visitors or the body's cells. If you have an autoimmune disorder, ask your doctor to test your vitamin D level. If you are deficient, your system might not be properly functioning.

Vitamin A

Vitamin A is valuable to our diets. It is called the anti-infective vitamin since it is needed for the immune system to function normally.

It can do this by maintaining the mucous cells that are barriers to germs that are trying to invade our bodies. It helps to produce white blood cells that are vital to our immune system.

Vitamin A is needed for the immune system, but large amounts are not needed. Your body can get vitamin A from animal or plant sources. It is necessary for the body to metabolize vitamin D effectively.

Vitamin B6

This vitamin group has functions within the immune system. People who are deficient in vitamin B6 have decreased the production of white blood cells and interleukin-2.

Balance is important with all B complex vitamins since many are interdependent. Just like vitamin A, you just need a little amount of B6. Your body does not make this vitamin, so a very healthy diet or supplements are needed to get it.

Antioxidants

These are a group of compounds that neutralize or destroy free radicals in the body. They protect against oxidative damage to cells that are caused by aging or exposure to toxic substances or pollutants.

Inflammation is common with autoimmune disease, but do not underestimate the problems of oxidative stress.

Within an immune response, the production of free radicals increases. This can cause oxidative stress. Most of the damage in autoimmune disease is caused by free radical damage to tissues and cell membranes.

Fish oil is a great supplement for people who suffer from an autoimmune disorder. Fish oil contains vitamin E that acts as an antioxidant when you combine it with selenium and vitamin C.

Antioxidants are found in healthy food like vegetables and fruits. The most effective ones are selenium, CoQ10, grape seed skin extract, beta-carotene, green tea extract, vitamin E, and vitamin C.

Fish oils contain omega-3 fatty acids like DHA and EPA. These can regulate the immune system.

These have been successful in helping conditions like rheumatoid arthritis, multiple sclerosis, lupus erythematosus, Crohn's disease, and arthritis.

DHEA

This is a pro-steroidal hormone that decreases as we age. A decrease in DHEA levels is linked to many degenerative and chronic disease like neurological functioning, stress disorders, depression, coronary artery disease, and cancer.

Immunity could have been compromised by poor regulation of cellular hormones that rule immune response due to the aging process.

A dietary approach is worth pursuing. There are many supplements out there and finding the right ones can be hard.

Always consult your doctor before deciding to take supplements to make sure none of them will react with your other medications that may have been prescribed to you. Investigate and explore your options.

Chapter 13: Exercise

Autoimmune diseases will throw your body off course. Your body is attacking its own tissues. What is normally good for you – like trying to boost the immune system – could actually make things worse. You will have to restrict eating foods that actually are nutrient dense and healthy. You cannot take anything for granted and have to think about and measure everything before you eat it. It may feel as if everything is a trigger.

Does this hold true for exercise as well? Do people who have been diagnosed with autoimmune diseases have to change how they train?

Exercise can actually help. You just need to learn to do it the right way or incur bad effects.

Try not to overtrain. Many autoimmune diseases have chronic inflammation. Whatever causes this inflammation to increase, like exercising too much, contributes to this pain. Overtraining will increase autoimmune symptoms because it increases your stress load.

Stay away from exercise that induces leaky gut. Intense, protracted exercise like 30 minutes of high-intensity metabolic workouts, 400-meter high-intensity intervals, long runs at race pace, all these will increase intestinal permeability. Leaky gut is linked to ankylosing spondylitis and rheumatoid arthritis. Researchers think it might play a role in hurting other autoimmune diseases, also.

Not exercising can make matters worse since it increases endorphins. Endorphins are actually what the body pumps out when it is trying to deal with pain and as a response to exercise. Exogenous opiates work through the endorphin receptor system. Endorphins play an important role in immune functions. Instead of diminishing or boosting it, endorphins will regulate immunity. They keep the system running smoothly. Without endorphins, the immune system will misbehave. Do this sound familiar?

Low Doses of Naltrexone or LDN is a good therapy for multiple sclerosis or another disease. It increases the endorphin secretions that will help regulate the system's behavior. Exercise is not as effective as LDN, but it does help.

It has the exact same relationship as everybody has when exercising. Too little is bad. Too much is bad. Recovery is a must. Intensity has to be balanced with the volume. When you have an autoimmune disease, the margin of error is a lot smaller.

What's the right way to exercise? It all depends on which autoimmune disease you have. Let's look at some common ones:

Rheumatoid Arthritis

This disease hurts. It makes exercise seem impossible. This is why many who have RA stay inactive. Exercise will help.

Exercise can improve functionality, reduce depression, and improve sleep. Acute exercise will keep cartilage from being destroyed and can help to thicken it.

What will work?

Yoga works. Many RA patients who did yoga regularly benefited from it. Yoga can reduce pain, improve function, and increase general well-being.

Light intensity activities work as well. Studies have shown that about five hours of light intensity activity every day was effective at improving cardiovascular health in RA patients instead of 35 minutes of moderate intensity training every day. This is not unique to RA; everyone can benefit from moving and walking for five hours instead of just jogging for 30 minutes.

Moving the painful joints works. For patients who have finger joint and hand pain, an exercise program that is centered on their hands can help improve functionality.

High-intensity activities will work. Four 4-minute high-intensity intervals on a bike exercise at 85 to 95 percent max rate can increase muscle mass and cardio fitness while reducing inflammatory markers for people who have RA. Patients could perform high-intensity aerobic and resistance training without having any issues.

Multiple Sclerosis

Just like RA, people who have multiple sclerosis can benefit from exercise. They begin to sleep better. If you begin early in life, you could reduce getting MS. Exercise increases brain-derived neurotrophic factors that are reduced in MS.

What works?

Tai Chi works. Tai chi improves functional outcomes in people who have MS.

Endurance and strength training work better together than alone. Doing a 24-week endurance and lifting program can increase BDNF (Brain-derived neurotrophic factor) in MS patients. A 12-week high-intensity and lifting program improved glucose tolerance.

Lifting during the morning works. Studies have shown that MS patients had less muscle strength and more muscle fatigue in the afternoons when compared to morning. Muscle oxidative capacity or the ability to burn fat did not change with times.

Intense exercise works. The higher the intensity, the more BDNF you make. BDNF is essential for creating and maintaining healthy neurons for a healthier brain.

Crohn's Disease

The body will attack the GI tract with Crohn's Disease. Since Crohn's could cause crippling GI pain, emergency diarrhea, joint pain, fatigue, and impaired digestion, many patients avoid exercise. Exercise can actually help a patient if they to overcome their mental roadblocks.

What will work?

Medium-intensity activities and short sprints work. Moderate cycling and all-out cycling were tolerated by children who have been diagnosed with Crohn's. In the moderate group, the markers were high. Another marker stayed elevated longer in the moderate group.

Aerobic and resistance training works. Both or alone will improve Crohn's symptoms by helping immune function.

Walking will work. A low-intensity walk three times each week will improve the quality of life for Crohn's patients.

Type-1 Diabetes

People forget about type-1 diabetes. This autoimmune disease attacks the pancreas and reduces the ability to make insulin. For patients that want to reduce how much insulin they inject, exercise is necessary.

What works?

Combining aerobic and resistance training works. This combination can lower insulin requirements and improve every marker of fitness as well as general feeling.

Resistance training works. Resistance training can lower blood glucose regardless of what intensity. Patients might need a dose of insulin after working out to keep glucose under control.

Lift heavy but keep it brief. High-intensity and low-volume short sprints like three to five rep sets. Intensity is relative so do not try to squat your bodyweight at first.

Spend the time on training on slow, long movements. Gardening walks, hikes, and gentle movements are the best. Anyone who has an autoimmune disease can do these.

Mobility training is needed with a disease that bothers joints and connective tissues. If the joints are compromised, other tissues need to be more mobile, loose, and limber.

Having an autoimmune disease will not make you fragile. You can still exercise if you give your body time to recover.

Find a Support Group

Having an autoimmune disease might leave you feeling isolated and alone. When you have finally processed the diagnosis, finding support from others might help you. Patients who have practical and emotional support during hard times have a handle on emotional health, improved health outcomes, and better quality of life.

If you do not like talking about your illness, you are not the only one. Most people find it hard to talk about their problems.

Why would you need support? You need support especially in the early stages, even if you just reach out to a couple of people. Here is why:

Support reduces stress: Talking about your feelings can reduce your stress. This is important since stress triggers symptoms for most.

Support will keep you on track: Having somebody to check in on you and see that you are taking your meds or eating right can help you control your illness.

You can get help faster in an emergency: If you have a health crisis at home or work, you will get through it if family or friends know how to help.

You will be more stable at work: Symptoms could occur at work and interfere with your job. Telling a co-worker or supervisor that you trust about what is going on can make it easier to continue working in spite of your illness.

How to Build a Support Team

There are many resources out there to help you when you have an illness. Try these:

Journal: You are the most important part of your support team. Write down your ideas, feelings, and thoughts. This is a good way to get rid of stress and plan other ways of communicating about the illness.

Reach out to friends and family: This needs to be your first stop. Be careful how you tell your loved one, so you do not overwhelm them. Do not whine. If you have a complaint, share it in a way to keep people listening.

Become a member of a faith community: For some, being a member of a faith community can give emotional benefits like stress reduction.

Join a support group: Talk to others who are coping with the same illness. They can give you invaluable emotional support and tips.

Go online: People who are limited or isolated with mobility can find help online. Some national foundations and societies support certain chronic illnesses.

Find help for depression: People who have a chronic illness often suffer from depression. Your doctor might prescribe an antidepressant to help with anxiety and depression. If you are feeling suicidal or overwhelmed, seek additional therapy. Depression is a reason to have a support group since isolation can contribute to depression.

Take time to nurture your illness: This will give you invaluable benefits for your emotional health.

Chapter 14: Motivation

If you have ever thought about ways you can stay healthy and fit, you may have realized that you are in serious need of motivation. It could be external or internal, but you must wake up each morning and stay motivated through the day and make the right choices when it comes to eating. The foods you eat will help you get through your workouts and will push you to the next level.

When struggling with any chronic illness, it is challenging to stay motivated, or you might be completely passionate. It just depends on your set of mind. Once you have been diagnosed with an autoimmune disease, you might think staying fit is impossible. Many people live the total opposite of healthy and fit. Not because their health problems prevented them from staying healthy and fit but mostly because they think negatively about their well-being.

This is not the case. Many people choose not to benefit from eating healthy and exercising to manage their disease. These people are just too lazy to care about their health. Staying fit is a challenge when you do not even feel like getting out of bed. Being fatigued is not anything to laugh at. It affects how you can handle your daily life.

So can you stay motivated, healthy, and fit when you have an autoimmune disease? Yes.

Begin each day with staying positive. It is hard to stay positive when you are in constant pain. Reminding yourself when you wake up that today is going to be a great day will help substantially.

Promise yourself that you are going to do one thing that your body will thank you for. Feel grateful that you will fight this disease with pride. This is easier when you are in remission. It can motivate you to get out of bed and choice a healthy food for breakfast or take a walk.

Make smart food choices. It is not easy to eat right when everybody around you is eating burgers and fries. Bad food is your enemy. Eating the wrong foods is the quickest way to flare up your condition. You have to be extremely smart about food choices. Learn your body and know what it can and cannot handle. If you do not want to wake up in pain the next day, make smart food choices today. This might seem too easy for people who want to be fit, but it is a true challenge for people with an autoimmune disease. One bad food choice can cause pain for weeks. Just don't do it. Learn to love your body and give it the food it needs and what it can handle.

You will fuse if you do not move. This is a great reminder for anyone who suffers from arthritis, but it holds true for any autoimmune disease. Just move. Your body is going to thank you. It does not have to be at an extremely intense movement. Just walk or do some low-intensity weight training a couple of times a week. Make sure you move. Try to do it for 30 minutes for about three or four days each week. When you begin to feel stronger, your body will amaze you on how it responds. You could get healthier from exercising alone, and it's great.

Know that you are going to have bad days. Do not get discouraged. There are going to be bad days. You will have days that you will not be able to eat or exercise right at all. The main thing here is to never give up. Accept that your body is going to win every now and then and you just need to listen to it and rest. Love yourself and learn to listen to your body. There will be other days that you can exercise. Tomorrow is just one day away. You will get active soon.

Learn to love your body. Listen to your body. Feed it with real, bountiful, and beautiful foods. Push it a bit so you can begin to feel better. Acknowledge and listen when you might be pushing it too far. Make health and fitness a priority and your body will begin thanking you.

Chapter 15: Food List

To help you get started in changing the way you eat to help your autoimmune disease, this chapter will provide you with a list of the best foods to consume.

Fruits and Vegetables

- All types of vegetables with lots of variety
- Colorful fruits and vegetables
- Cruciferous vegetables
- Sea vegetables – excluding algae
- Watercress
- Turnips
- Mustard greens
- Kale
- Cabbage
- Brussels sprouts
- Broccoli
- Arugula

Fruits and Vegetables to Avoid

- Tomatillos
- Tamarillos
- Potatoes – sweet potatoes
- Pimentos

- Pepinos
- Paprika
- Naranjillas
- Kutjera
- Hot peppers – habanero jalapenos
- Goji berries
- Garden huckleberry
- Eggplant
- Cocona
- Capsicum
- Cape gooseberry
- Bush tomato
- Ashwagandha

Protein

- Glycine-rich foods
- Fish and shellfish
- Offal and organ meat
- Wild boar
- Venison
- Turkey – in moderation
- Rabbit

- Pork
- Pheasant – in moderation
- Lamb
- Elk
- Duck – in moderation
- Chicken – in moderation
- Buffalo
- Beef

Fats

- Olives
- Animal fats
- Fatty fish
- Coconut
- Avocados

Probiotics

- Water and coconut milk kefir
- Kombucha
- Fermented fruits and veggies
- Coconut milk yogurt

Spices and herbs

- Turmeric

- Thyme
- Tarragon
- Spearmint
- Savory leaves
- Salt
- Sage
- Saffron
- Rosemary
- Peppermint
- Parsley
- Oregano leaves
- Onion powder
- Marjoram leaves
- Mace
- Lavender
- Horseradish
- Ginger
- Garlic
- Dill weed
- Cloves
- Cinnamon

- Coriander
- Chives
- Chervil
- Chamomile
- Bay leaves
- Basil
- Lemon balm

Spices and Herbs to eat in moderation

- White pepper
- Vanilla bean
- Star anise
- Pink peppercorns
- Juniper
- Green peppercorns
- Cardamom
- Caraway
- Black pepper
- Allspice

Spices and herbs to avoid

- Sesame seed
- Poppy seed

- Paprika
- Nutmeg
- Mustard seed
- Fenugreek
- Fennel seed
- Dill seed
- Cumin seeds
- Curry
- Coriander seeds
- Chili powder
- Chili pepper flakes
- Celery seeds
- Cayenne
- Black caraway
- Annatto seed
- Anise seed

Other foods that need to be avoided

- Seeds – seed-based spices, coffee, cocoa
- Nuts
- NSAIDs – ibuprofen or aspirin
- Non-nutritive sweeteners – stevia

- Fructose – no more than 20g each day
- Food additives
- Thickeners and emulsifiers
- Eggs – especially the whites
- Alcohol

Foods which cross-react with gluten

- Teff
- Tapioca
- Soy
- Spelt
- Sorghum
- Sesame
- Rye
- Rice
- Quinoa
- Potato
- Polish wheat
- Oats
- Milk
- Millet
- Hemp

- Corn
- Coffee – imported, espresso, latte, instant
- Chocolate
- Buckwheat
- Barley
- amaranth

For the grains, you can select what kind of grain you want. But always remember, when selecting a food, you should go by how certain food makes you feel. You may be able to eat something that another person cannot. This is just a guideline; the important thing is just to get to know you.

PART 1.5:

Meal plan and recipes

Chapter 16: Meal Plan

To help get you started with your autoimmune diet, in this section, you will find a one-week meal plan and the recipes that correspond with it. These are fun and tasty recipes, and an extremely easy meal plan to stick to. You will be making most of what you will eat all week on Sunday. One recipe, the Bacon-Beef Liver Pate is for snack during the week. Let's get started.

Sunday:

- Breakfast: Italian-Spiced 50/50 Sausages
- Lunch: Cabbage and Avocado Salad
- Dinner: Citrus and Herb Pot Roast and Rainbow Roasted Root Vegetables

Monday:

- Breakfast: Three-Herb Beef Patties
- Lunch: Citrus and Herb Pot Roast and Rainbow Roasted Root Vegetables
- Dinner: Citrus and Herb Pot Roast and Cabbage and Avocado Salad

Tuesday:

- Breakfast: Italian-Spiced 50/50 Sausages
- Lunch: Citrus and Herb Pot Roast and Rainbow Roasted Root Vegetables
- Dinner: Ginger-Baked Salmon and Beet and Fennel Salad

Wednesday:

- Breakfast: Three-Herb Beef Patties
- Lunch: Ginger Baked Salmon and Beet and Fennel Salad
- Dinner: Carrot and Sweet Potato Chili

Thursday:

- Breakfast: Italian-Spiced 50/50 Sausages
- Lunch: Carrot and Sweet Potato Chili
- Dinner: Sear-Roasted Pork Chops and Early Spring Salad

Friday:

- Breakfast: Three-Herb Beef Patties
- Lunch: Sear-Roasted Pork Chops and Early Spring Salad
- Dinner: Carrot and Sweet Potato Chili

Saturday:

- Breakfast: Italian-Spiced 50/50 Sausages
- Lunch: Carrot and Sweet Potato Chili
- Dinner: Garlic Mayo Shredded Chicken Breast Curried Chicken Salad

Cabbage and Avocado Salad

Ingredients:

2 cubed avocados

3 tsp. salt

2 tsp. coconut vinegar

4 tbsps. olive oil

2 blood oranges, juiced

1 handful parsley, chopped

3 carrots, grated

1 small red onion, sliced

1 head cabbage, shredded

Instructions:

Toss together the carrots, onion, cabbage, and most of the parsley.

Mix the salt, coconut vinegar, olive oil, and the orange juice.

Pour the dressing over the vegetables and toss together.

Add the remaining parsley and the avocado on top.

Citrus and Herb Pot Roast

Ingredients:

Fresh herbs

2 parsnips, chunked

3 carrots, chunked

1 bay leaf

1 orange, juiced

2 tbsps. Apple Cider Vinegar (ACV)

¾ c bone broth

1 ½ tsps. salt

2-3 lbs. roast

1 tbsp. coconut oil

Instructions:

Your oven should be at 300 F. Add the coconut oil into a Dutch oven and then place in the roast and brown it on all sides. Turn the heat off and take the roast out of the pot and salt it.

Place the bay leaf, orange juice, cider vinegar, and bone broth into the pot. Place the roast back in and surround it with the parsnips and carrots. Add a generous sprinkling of the fresh herbs over everything.

Cover the pot with a lid and place it in the oven for two to three hours. Make sure that you check to make sure there is enough liquid in the pot every now and then. Once cooked, pull the meat apart with some forks and enjoy.

Rainbow Roasted Root Vegetables

Ingredients:

1 tsp. salt

3 tbsps. coconut oil

2 parsnips, chunked

3 carrots, chunked

1 turnip, chunked

4 beets, chunked

Instructions:

Your oven should be at 400 F. Mix together the parsnip, carrots, turnip, and beets together and place them on a baking sheet. Sprinkle with some salt and drizzle with some melted coconut oil.

Place them in the oven and cook for 45 to 60 minutes. Make sure you stir every 20 minutes so that everything becomes tender and caramelized.

Ginger Baked Salmon

Ingredients:

3 tbsps. parsley, minced

¼ tsp. sea salt

¼ tsp. ginger

2 tbsps. melted coconut oil

16/24 oz. salmon fillet

Instructions:

Your oven should be at 400 F. Clean your salmon and place it onto an oiled baking sheet. Rush the coconut oil over the fillet and sprinkle it with sea salt and ginger. Place in the oven for 15 to 20 minutes.

Beet and Fennel Salad

Ingredients:

Dressing:

¼ tsp. salt

1 minced garlic clove

½ lemon, juiced

1 tbsp. ACV

½ c olive oil

Salad:

Sprig mint, chopped

Handful parsley, chopped

1 fennel bulb

1 cucumber

4 beets

Instructions

Mix all of the dressing ingredients in a bowl. Slice up the fennel, beets, and cucumber very thinly. Add them to a large bowl and toss them together with the dressing.

Carrot and Sweet Potato Chili

Ingredients:

Cilantro

1-2 avocados

2 lbs. ground beef

1 tsp. salt

4 c bone broth

4 c sweet potatoes, chunked

2 c carrots, chunked

1 tbsp. thyme

8 minced garlic cloves

1 onion, chopped

2 tbsps. coconut oil

Instructions:

Melt the coconut oil in a large pot. Place in the onion and allow to cook until soft, and then mix in the thyme and garlic, cooking for a few more minutes.

Place in the sweet potato and carrot and let them cook for about five minutes. Pour in the salt and the bone broth and allow it to come to a boil. Place on the lid and let cook for 20 minutes. Veggies should be soft.

Add in the ground beef and mix. Let it cook for another 15 minutes. Serve with a slice of avocado and cilantro.

Italian-spiced 50/50 sausages

Ingredients:

1 tbsp. coconut oil

½ tsp. salt

½ tsp. garlic powder

1 tbsp. minced parsley

1 tbsp. minced thyme

1 tbsp. minced oregano

1 lb. ground pork

1 lb. ground beef

Instructions:

Add all of the ingredients, except for the oil, in a bowl and mix them with your hands until well combined. Form the meat into eight to ten patties. You can freeze them now by placing wax paper between the patties and sliding them into a freezer safe bag or container.

When you are ready to eat, melt the oil and fry them for 10 minutes per side.

Three-Herb Beef Patties

Ingredients:

1 tbsp. coconut oil

1 tsp. salt

1 tbsp. sage

1 tbsp. thyme

1 tbsp. rosemary

2 lbs. ground beef

Instructions:

Mix all of the herbs, beef, and salt together with your hands. Form them into patties. At this point, they can be frozen with wax paper between the patties.

Once ready to cook them, heat the oil in a skillet and fry for about five to eight minutes on each side.

Bacon-Beef Liver Pate

Ingredients:

1/2 tsp. salt

½ c melted coconut oil

2 tbsps. thyme, minced

2 tbsps. rosemary, minced

1 lb. beef liver

4 minced garlic cloves

1 onion, minced

6 pcs. bacon

Instructions:

Cook the bacon until it is crisp and allow to cool. Place the onion in the bacon grease and let cook for two minutes. Mix in the garlic and add the liver. Sprinkle everything with herbs and let cook for three to five minutes or until cooked through.

Turn the heat off and add everything to a blender and mix with the coconut oil and salt until it turns into a paste.

Cut the bacon up and stir it into the plate.

Sear-Roasted Pork Chops

Ingredients:

1 tbsp. coconut oil

1 tsp. salt

2 tbsps. fresh herbs

2 pork chops

Instructions:

Your oven should be at 350 F. Mix the salt and herbs together. Add oil to a pan, and then rub the herbs over the chops.

Once the pan is hot, sear the chops for a couple of minutes on each side. Slide them into the oven for ten minutes.

Early Spring Salad

Ingredients:

1 fennel bulb, sliced

1 grapefruit, sectioned

4 c arugula

¼ tsp. salt

¼ tsp. ginger

1 tbsp. ACV

1 lemon, juiced

¼ c EVOO

Instructions:

Add the salt, ginger, vinegar, lemon juice, and olive oil in a bowl and mix well.

Add the all the other ingredients into the bowl and toss together. Toss with the dressing just before serving.

Garlic Mayo

Ingredients:

¼ tsp. salt

3-4 garlic cloves

¼ c EVOO

½ c warm water

½ c coconut concentrate, warmed

Instructions:

Place the salt, garlic, olive oil, water, and coconut in a blender and mix until the sauce thickens.

Allow this to cool to room temp.

Curried Chicken Salad

Ingredients:

2 tbsps. parsley, chopped

¼ c raisins

¼ c chopped onion

1 lb. chicken breast, cooked and shredded

¼ tsp. salt

1 tsp. ginger

2 tsp. turmeric

½ lemon, juiced

1 tsp. ACV

½ c garlic mayo

Instructions:

Whisk together the salt, ginger, turmeric, lemon juice, vinegar, and mayo. Mix in the raisins, onion, and chicken. Serve with some parsley.

PART 2

Chapter 1: What is Inflammation Anyway?

Did you know that inflammation is actually a good thing as long as it is limited in duration? Inflammation is the body's natural response to infection or injury. As the immune system begins working, minor inflammation is evidenced by the five universal signs: redness, warmth, swelling, pain in the injured area and unable to function. When inflammation becomes excessive, it begins to work against the healthy cells erroneously, which can lead to disease and pain.

Most people are familiar with inflammation after an injury. For example, a ballet dancer loses her balance and sprains her ankle. She notices the injured limb swelling and turning red. Upon touching the skin, it is warm to touch and there is quite a bit of noticeable pain. Finally, the dancer is unable to complete her routine because she is unable to continue to use her ankle and must have assistance with walking. This is inflammation in its normal state. This is what inflammation is supposed to do. Unfortunately, it doesn't always function properly. That's when inflammation becomes a problem.

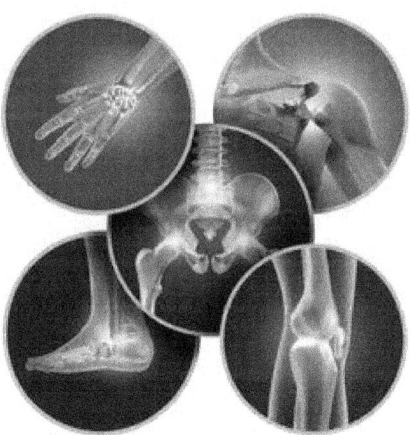

When the body's tissue experiences bad stimuli, it responds in a complicated fashion with several parts including pathogens, irritants, or damaged cells and inflammation. Inflammation is the protector of the group and gets the help of immune cells, molecular mediators, and blood vessels. Inflammation's job is to eradicate the original reason for cell injury, eliminate neurotic cells and tissues that were damaged by the cause of the stimuli and subsequent inflammatory process, and begin fixing the tissue.

Inflammation is categorized into 2 types: acute and chronic. Acute inflammation is what we mentioned before: the initial response of the body towards the damaging stimuli. It is achieved by plasma and leukocytes moving around more from the blood to the damaged tissues. Chronic inflammation is basically just prolonged inflammation. That is the inflammation that causes problems for the overall health of the person.

Chapter 2: Inflammation causes what?

As mentioned before, inflammation is the normal process in which the body creates and sends out white blood cells to cleanse and annihilate alien matter in the bloodstream. When constant stress from external conditions or dwelling on past stressful events for extended periods of time, the levels of c-reactive protein elevates and creates chronic inflammation.

Chronic inflammation is detrimental to the body and can be the cause or the agitator of many chronic health conditions and it affects all areas of the body. In the gut, inflammation can cause Inflammatory Bowel Disease (IBD) which comes in a couple forms: Ulcerative Colitis and Chron's Disease.

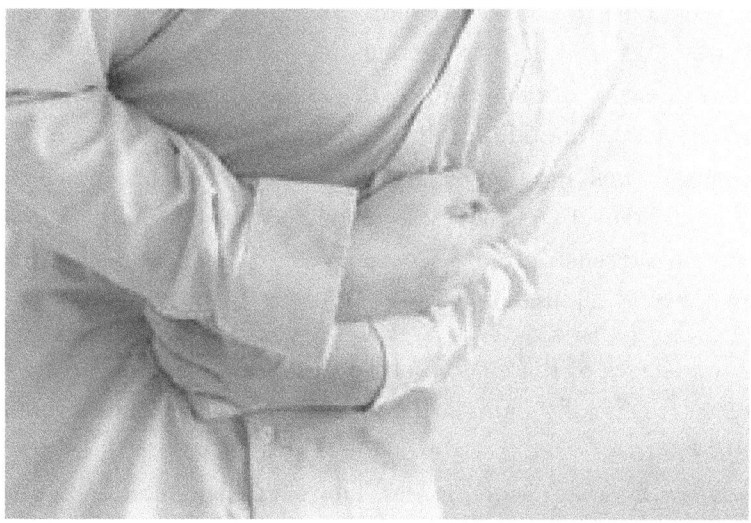

Inflammatory Bowel Disease is a broad term that describes the disorders that require chronic inflammation of the digestive tract and can be crippling and can have potentially deadly complications. *Ulcerative colitis* is the cause for chronic inflammation and ulcers in the innermost lining of the colon (large intestine) and rectum. *Chron's disease* is the inflammation of the lining of the digestive tract and it frequently spreads will into affected tissues. IBD symptoms are varied depending on the location and the severity of the inflammation and may range from mild to severe. Symptoms common to both Chron's disease and ulcerative colitis include:

- Diarrhea
- Unintended weight loss
- Abdominal cramping and pain
- Reduced appetite
- Blood in your stool
- Fever and fatigue

Probably the most commonly recognized area to be affected are the joints. Rheumatoid Arthritis (RA) is an ongoing inflammatory disorder of the joints. RA affects more than simply the joints. It can sometimes damage the skin, heart and blood vessels, eyes, and lungs. Rheumatoid arthritis causes painful swelling and the effects can, over time, cause bone to erode and joints to deform. Sadly, despite new types of medication greatly improving treatment options, severe cases of rheumatoid arthritis still cause major physical disabilities.

In the early stages of rheumatoid arthritis, it is the smaller joints that feel the effects. It generally starts in the joints that connect the fingers to the hand and the toes to the feet. Over time, the disease symptoms spread to the elbows, wrists, shoulders, ankles, knees, and shoulders. The majority of the time, the symptoms occur in the same joints on both sides of the body. The usual signs and symptoms of rheumatoid arthritis are:

- Fatigue, fever, weight loss
- Tender, warm, swollen joints
- Stiffness in the joints (usually worse after inactivity and in the mornings)

About 40% of RA sufferers will have signs and symptoms of non-joint structures being affected:

- Kidneys
- Eyes
- Blood Vessels
- Nerve Tissue
- Lungs
- Bone Marrow
- Heart
- Salivary glands

Rheumatoid arthritis symptoms are fluid and will come and go. Flare-ups, times when the disease is more active, alternate with times of brief relief from the symptoms. Long-term effects may cause joints to move out of place and become deformed.

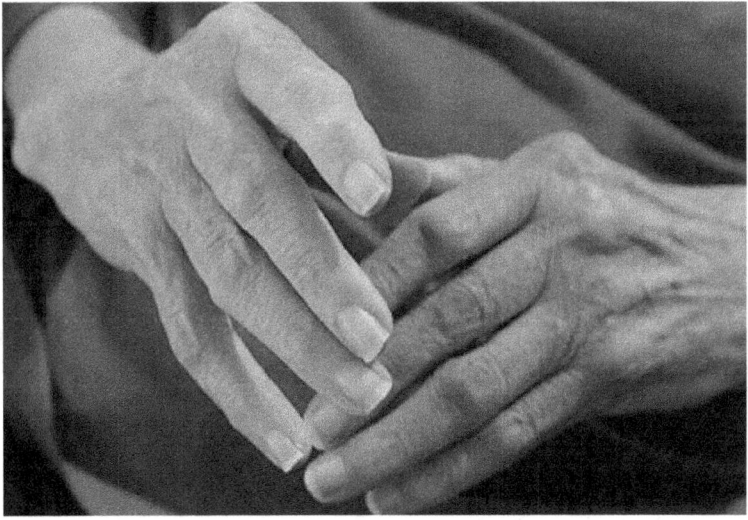

Another area of the body that can be adversely affected by chronic inflammation is the heart. Myocarditis is the inflammation of the actual heart muscle (a.k.a. myocardium) and can affect not only the muscle itself but also its vitally important electrical system. If the electrical system goes haywire, then the heart is not as able to pump and the result is rapid or abnormal heart rhythms (a.k.a. arrhythmias). The usual culprit that causes myocarditis is a viral infection, but it has been known to be the result of a reaction to a medication or simply a very general inflammatory condition. Severe myocarditis is potentially very harmful to your overall health. It weakens the heart to the point that the remainder of the body is unable to receive adequate amounts of blood. Over time, clots can form in the heart that left unchecked could result in a stroke or heart attack.

Because of how serious the consequences of this inflammatory disease, it is of great importance to know the symptoms of myocarditis and to take action at the earliest signs. Mild cases or very early on, there may be no symptoms or mild ones—say, some chest pain or shortness of breath. On the more serious cases, the symptoms and signs do vary depending on the actual cause of the disease. Symptoms and telltale signs to watch for are:

- Shortness of breath (no matter if actively doing something or resting)
- Swelling of ankles, feet, or legs with fluid retention
- Chest pain
- Arrhythmias (abnormal or rapid heart rhythms)
- Fatigue
- Various other symptoms and signs conducive to a viral infection (a headache, body aches, sore throat, diarrhea, joint pain, or fever)

Children who develop myocarditis may have different distinct symptoms:

- Arrhythmias (abnormal or rapid heart rhythms)
- Breathing difficulties
- Rapid breathing

- Fainting
- Fever

Another common condition that gets attention is not readily acquainted with inflammation among the general population conversation. This surprise condition is psoriasis. The common skin condition accelerates the life cycle of skins, thus causing skin cells to quickly layer up on top of each other. The resulting additional skin cells form painful and itchy red scaly patches. Like other inflammatory conditions, psoriasis comes and goes often. While there is no current cure for the chronic condition, the main treatment goal is to slow the growth of skin cells. Lifestyle changes (managing stress, cease smoking, applying moisturizers) may help with the uncomfortable symptoms:

- Swollen and stiff joints
- Dry and cracking skin that may bleed
- Red patches of skin covered with thick silver-colored scales
- Soreness, burning, or itching
- Pitted, ridged, or thickened nails
- Small spots that scale (especially in children)

Majority of the types of psoriasis go through flare-up cycles that can be for weeks at a time to months in a row. The flare-ups may be followed by a period of easing up or even complete remission.

There are actually several different types of psoriasis including Plaque, Nail, Guttate, Inverse, Pustular Erythrodermic, and Psoriatic Arthritis. They cover just about every area of the body and each has their own set of symptoms and discomforts.

Although the scientific community is still researching, there have been some studies that suggest that inflammation has a role in cancer. Harvard University conducted a study in 2014 that suggested the risk of colorectal cancer was possibly higher if the body had inflammation. The results concluded that obese teenagers with high levels of inflammation had a 63% greater risk of developing colorectal cancer during adulthood. However, their many variables of the study subjects made it unrealistic to make a definite claim. The Mayo Clinic states that gene mutations that occur after birth are not inherited and can be caused by a number of possible outside forces including radiation, viruses, smoking, carcinogens, hormones, lack of exercise, obesity, and of course chronic inflammation.

Inflammation causes less serious negative effects as well such as sabotaging sleep. In 2009, Case Western Reserve University conducted a study in which people reported less or more sleep than average had elevated levels of inflammation-related proteins in their systems. Paradoxically, insufficient sleep can cause an increase of inflammation and fluid buildup.

Chronic inflammation is bad for the lungs as well. The results are infections, asthma and COPD (emphysema and chronic bronchitis). Both asthma and any version of COPD cause shortness of breath and limits the daily activities of a person resulting in a quality of life that may be less than desirable.

Periodontitis is an infection of gums. This is a seriously damaging condition. Damage is done to the soft tissue and the bone supporting your teeth gets destroyed. Periodontitis can loosen teeth or lead to absolute loss of teeth. The good news is this infection is very preventable and treatable. The initial treatment is a recommendation the person works on improving oral hygiene by brushing twice a day, daily flossing, and getting regular dental checkups. If the gums are firm and pale pink fitting snuggly around each tooth, they are indeed healthy. If the following symptoms are present, they are indicative of periodontitis and an exam and treatment by a dentist is highly recommended. Signs and symptoms to look for are:

- Painful chewing
- Bad breath
- Easy to bleed gums

- Tender-to-touch gums
- Swollen or puffy gums
- Bright red, purplish, or dusky red gums
- Gums that recede making your teeth to appear longer than normal
- Pus between teeth and gums
- Loose teeth
- Spaces developing between teeth and gums
- Changes in how your teeth fit when biting

Like Psoriasis, there are several typed of periodontitis with three being the most common: *Chronic*, *Aggressive*, and *Necrotizing periodontal disease*. Chronic periodontitis is the most common, caused by plaque buildup and has a slow deterioration that, over time, improves and worsens but will cause destruction if left untreated. Aggressive periodontitis onsets in childhood or early adulthood. It tends to be a hereditary trait causing quick disintegration of bone and loss of teeth if not treated. Necrotizing periodontal disease generally occurs in people with weakened immune systems (HIV, cancer, or other causes) and malnutrition.

Other problems associated with inflammatory conditions are bone damage and depression. The inflammation can prevent bone-building nutrients being absorbed such as calcium and vitamin D. Chronic inflammation can be linked to depression as well and is responsible for depressive symptoms such as low mood, poor sleep, and lack of appetite.

With all these negative effects of inflammation, it is important to understand what inflammation is, what conditions it causes or aggravates, and how to treat it. Once inflammation is understood, then steps can be taken to prevent, treat, or eliminate the chronic inflammation. One important step to take is making lasting lifestyle changes such as choosing an anti-inflammatory diet plan to follow.

Chapter 3: Which Diet plan Works for you?

So the inflammation is in there, now what? First and foremost, seeking and following the advice of your primary care physician is crucial to proper treatment. He or she is already familiar with your medical history and lifestyle. They can make recommendations that are custom-made for your situation. Most likely, the first recommendation of any physician will be mild to moderate lifestyle changes depending on the type and severity of the inflammation. The first step to take is changing up dietary behaviors. Thankfully, with the heightened awareness and celebrities trying every diet out there, the common population has several diet plans to choose from—many of which have anti-inflammatory tendencies.

Dr. Weil's Anti-Inflammatory Diet is currently one with some popularity. It is not a weight loss plan. However, it is possible and perhaps likely that some minimal weight loss can occur. It is rather a strategic plan for choosing and preparing foods that have anti-inflammatory properties. The selections are chosen based on scientific knowledge on how they can assist the body to maintain ideal health.

Dr. Andrew Weil, a Harvard medicine graduate, is a best-selling author, internal medicine instructor and the framer and director of the University of Arizona in Tucson's Program of Integrative Medicine (PIM), which he founded back in 1994. He informs and gives insight on how to use traditional and complementary medicine techniques to utilize fully the body's natural healing mechanics.

Dr. Weil's anti-inflammatory diet plan is based on a foundation of plant-based foods with a recommendation of eating 4-5 vegetables and 3-4 fruits a day. From there, he uses a pyramid formation for the distribution of other food categories. Unlike the USDA recommended food pyramid with only 6 sections, Weil's pyramid has 15 sections. The detailed pyramid may seem daunting at first, but if it is looked at as an illustration of the entire diet plan, then it becomes easier to understand.

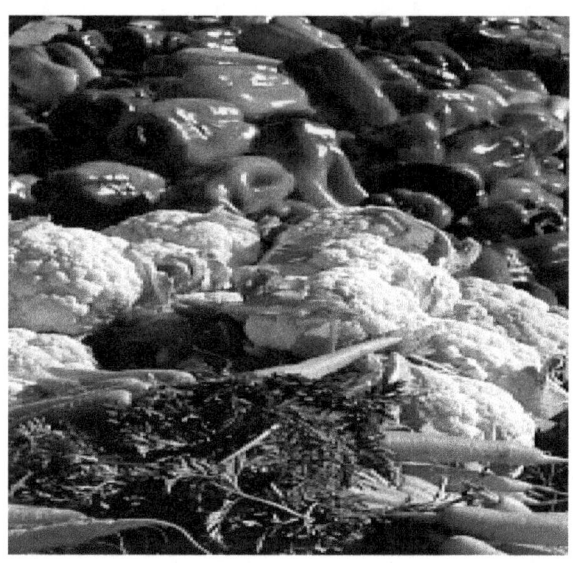

Fruits and vegetables are the foundation of the plan. It is recommended to eat organic or local produce is chosen over imported. The next row is made up of up to 5 servings per day of whole or cracked grains, 3 servings per week of pasta, 2 servings per day of legumes and beans. Next are friendly fats: extra-virgin olive oil, nuts, avocados, and seeds (5-7 servings per day). The fourth row emphasizes consuming omega-3 rich fish and shellfish (2-6 times a week). The next row recommends 1-2 servings per day of tofu, edamame, and other whole soy products. Above that row are cooked Asian mushrooms. The benefits of the fungi must be phenomenal because the dieter is permitted to eat unlimited amounts of this one food type. Above them in smaller amounts are other sources of protein. Finally, the top 5 categories are: healthy herbs and spices (in unlimited amounts), tea (white or oolong, 2-4 cups per day), supplemental vitamins (daily), healthy sweets such as dark chocolate (very sparingly) and if any alcohol is consumed, it should be red wine with less than 1-2 glasses a day.

Dr. Weil's plan, although rather specific, is simple in idea. Basically, avoid all processed foods. Soda and junk food are filled with artificial flavors and colors, and the chemicals used to create them are oftentimes conducive to inflammation rather than reducing it. Look for his diet plan books online and at your favorite bookstore.

The Mediterranean diet (a.k.a. arthritis diet) is an excellent anti-inflammatory diet plan. Many physicians nowadays are recommending it to their arthritis patients. The Mediterranean diet allows minimal amounts of bad fats and non-organic foods while encouraging consuming an abundance of vegetables, fish, fruits, beans, as well as nuts. The diet receives praises for its anti-aging and disease-fighting abilities.

Possible outcomes after eating these foods could include:

- Curbing inflammation (easing arthritis)
- Protection against chronic conditions (cancer, stroke, and more)
- Potential weight loss (great for joint pain)
- Lower blood pressure
- Happier joints and heart

Most anti-inflammatory plans share similar food suggestions: fish, nuts and seeds, fruits and veggies, olive oil, beans, and whole grains. The recommendations are in line with the Arthritis Foundation.

In 2004, a study revealed that those who consumed the higher amounts of omega-3 had lower levels of interleukin-6 and C-reactive protein, both of which have been connected to inflammation. The sea offers a vast supply of cold-water fish. Taking 600–1,000 mg of fish oil supplements can reduce swelling, pain, joint stiffness, and tenderness.

Eating 1.5 ounces of nuts daily (approximately a handful) reduces your chances of dying from inflammatory illnesses more than those who ate fewer nuts. One possible reason why is because nuts contain vitamin B6 which helps reduce inflammatory markers.

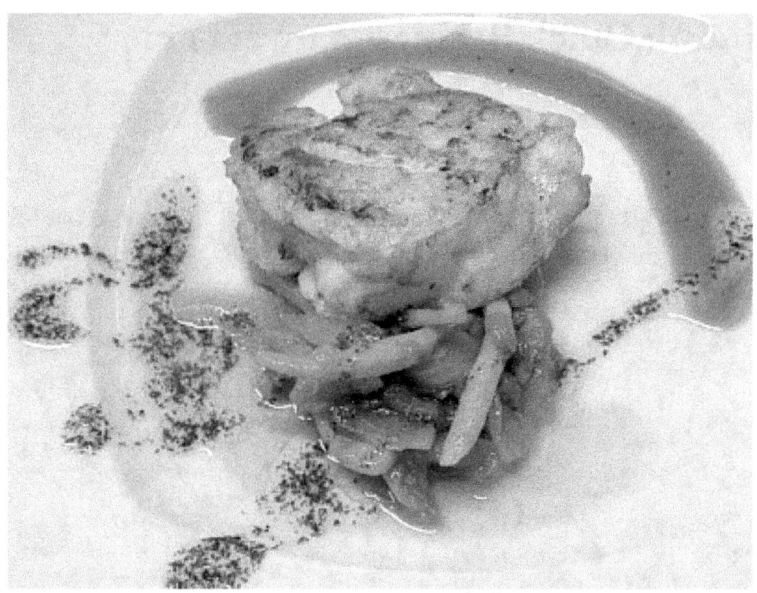

For modern dieters, there are apps such as Noom. Noom assigns the users a personal registered dietician. Noom is free to download the basic features on both iTunes and Google Play Store. Apple iTunes has the IF Tracker app that helps users find anti-inflammatory foods and build a healthy anti-inflammatory diet. Its list of over 2,000 generic and brand name foods track calories, fat, protein, calcium, potassium, sodium, cholesterol, carbs, and fiber.

Chapter 4: Quick Recipes to try at home

Probably the fastest sabotage of any diet is time. In this extremely fast-paced world, we need to maximize our time, and having quick meal ideas is a great place to start. In this chapter are recipes that are great to eat to reduce inflammation yet not take up a ton of time.

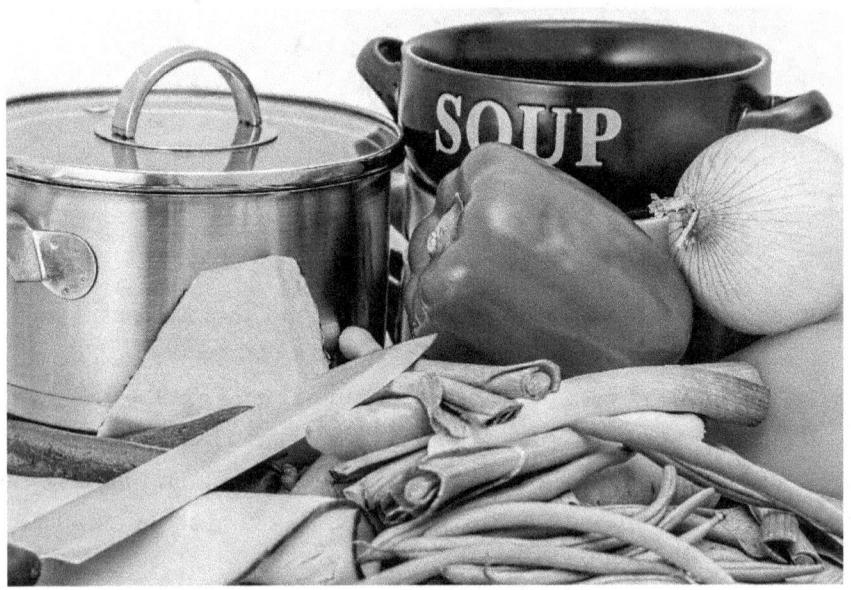

Chickpea and Vegetable Coconut Curry

Feeds 4. Time to the table: 30 minutes.

Ingredients:

    4 scallions, sliced thinly

    ¼ cup chopped fresh cilantro

    Steamed rice (optional)

    1 can (28oz) cooked chickpeas

    1 ½ cup frozen peas

Salt and ground pepper

1 lime cut in half

1 small head cauliflower (bite sized pieces)

1 can (14 oz) coconut milk

1 thinly sliced red bell pepper

1 tsp coriander

2 tsp chili powder

1 Tbsp extra-virgin olive oil

1 Tbsp minced fresh ginger

3 Tbsp red curry paste

3 minced garlic cloves

1 thinly sliced red onion

Directions:

Step 1: Heat olive oil! Pour into a large pot heat over medium heat. Sauté the slices of bell pepper approximately 4–5 minutes. Stir in the garlic and ginger, continue sautéing.

Step 2: Next, add the bite-sized cauliflower and toss well. Stir in the chili powder, red curry paste, and coriander. Cook until the whole mixture is slightly dark (about 1 minute).

Step 3: Stir in the coconut milk and simmer over a medium-low heat. Cover the pot and continue simmering until the cauliflower is tender (approximately 8–10 minutes).

Step 4: Remove the lid and squeeze lime juice into the curry, stirring to combine well. Add the peas and chickpeas, season with pepper and salt, then bring the mixture back to a simmer.

Step 5: Serve with rice (optional) and garnish each portion with 1 tbsp cilantro and 1 tbsp scallions.

White Turkey Chili Avocado

Serves: 8

    1 diced avocado

    1 can white beans (15 oz.)

    1 can (15 oz.) kernel corn

    4 cups chicken broth

    1 lb. ground turkey

    2 tsp ground cumin

    1 tsp ground coriander

    Salt & Pepper

    2 Tbsp extra-virgin olive oil

    1 diced onion (large)

    Minced garlic cloves (4)

    1 tsp pepper (cayenne)

Directions:

Step 1: Heat olive oil! Place in a large pot and heat to medium heat. Toss in the onion, cook until the onion is tender and clear looking (approximately 6–8 minutes). Stir in the garlic and sauté about 1 more minute.

Step 2: Add the turkey meat and brown until fully cooked (about 5–7 minutes). Once it is fully cooked, add the cayenne, cumin, and coriander, and then add salt and pepper to taste. Cook the seasoned meat until the aroma teases your senses (about 1–2 minutes).

Step 3: Add the broth and simmer over medium heat. Turn down the heat to low and simmer 30 to 35 minutes.

Step 4: Stir in the beans and corn, simmer for 2–3 minutes.

Serve by ladling into your favorite bowls then top with 1–2 tablespoons avocado and serve immediately.

Chicken and Snap Pea Stir Fry

Serves: 4   Prep Time: Approximately 20 minutes

Ingredients

1 bunch of thinly sliced scallions

1 thinly sliced red bell pepper

1 ¼ cup thinly sliced, boneless, skinless chicken breast

2 minced garlic cloves

2 tbsp rice vinegar

2 tbsp Sriracha (optional)

2 tbsp (plus extra for topping) sesame seeds

2 ½ cups snap peas

3 tbsp soy sauce

3 tbsp (plus extra for topping) fresh chopped cilantro

Directions:

Step 1: Heat the oil in a large sauté pan using medium heat. Next, toss in the garlic with the scallions and continue cooking until just tender (approximately 1 minute). Add the snap peas and bell pepper to the mixture. Continue sautéing for 2 to 3 minutes until slightly tender.

Step 2: Place the sliced chicken breasts in the pan with the mixture and cook until fully cooked and golden in color and the vegetables are tender. (approximately 4–5 minutes)

Step 3: Once the chicken is fully cooked and the vegetables are completely tender, add the rice vinegar, Sriracha (optional), and sesame seeds then toss the mixture well to combine. Simmer for an additional 1–2 minutes.

Step 4: Stir in the cilantro and garnish with a sprinkle of sesame seeds and cilantro.

Serve immediately for best taste.

Greek Turkey Burgers with Tzatziki Sauce

Serves: 4

Ingredients

¼ tsp red pepper flakes

½ tsp dried oregano

½ fresh parsley chopped

¾ cup of bread crumbs

1 minced sweet onion

1 egg

1 Tbsp extra-virgin olive oil

ground turkey (approx. 1 lb)

Fresh ground pepper and salt

Tzatziki Sauce

¼ cup fresh parsley, chopped

½ cucumber diced

1 pinch of garlic powder

1 cup yogurt

1 tbsp extra-virgin olive oil

2 tbsp lemon juice

Salt and black pepper

Toppings

½ red onion, sliced

2 sliced tomatoes

4 whole-wheat hamburger buns

8 lettuce leaves

Directions

Step 1: Preheat the olive oil using a small skillet then add the minced onion. After 3–4 minutes, add the garlic and sauté for an additional minute. Set that mixture aside to permit it to cool.

Step 2: Combine in a medium bowl an egg, parsley, oregano, red-pepper flakes and ground turkey with the onion mixture. Add the bread crumbs to the bowl and then season with salt and pepper. Stir well.

Step 3: While waiting for the oven to preheat to 375F, divide the mixture into 4 equal patties. Generously apply non-stick cooking spray to a large oven-safe skillet pre-heat it with a medium-high heat.

Step 4: Cook the patties in the skillet until each is seared on both sides (approximately 4–5 minutes each side). Place the pan in the warm oven to complete the cooking of the burgers (approximately 15 to 17 minutes).

Step 5: While they are cooking, make the Tzatziki Sauce. In a medium bowl, combine the cucumber, olive oil lemon juice and garlic powder with the yogurt. Salt and pepper to your taste preference then mix in the parsley.

Step 6: Toast the buns if desired and then add each patty to the bottom bun. To the top, add ¼ cup of the tzatziki, 2 leaves of lettuce, 2 slices of tomato, then the top half of the bun. Serve immediately.

Conclusion

Inflammation is a very normal part of everybody. It is a natural response to a traumatic event on a person. Normally, the inflammation does its job then it goes away. When it doesn't go away, then it becomes chronic. Chronic inflammation is detrimental to a person's health and, if left unchecked, has serious and even sometimes fatal consequences.

It is very important to visit your doctor and together create a plan of treatments. Carefully consider the many prescription medications available and discuss possible lifestyle changes. One of the easiest and quickest lifestyle changes is choosing new food to eat. This book described different diet plans. Any of the anti-inflammatory diet plans are ideal for lowering chronic inflammation and reducing the complications from it.

Whether you prefer a paperback or hardback book to guide you or you choose one of the many apps available, the fundamentals are the same. The principles behind the anti-inflammatory diet have been proven to reduce inflammation and bring relief to sufferers.

Diets that reduce inflammation doesn't necessarily mean they are bland and boring. There are many recipes that are not only tasty but also quick. Check out the many different websites that offer resources and recipes; the Arthritis Foundation is a great place to start. Always be sure to check with your physician for all your healthcare decisions. He or she may be able to refer you to a licensed dietician who can custom tailor a diet for you that meets all your nutritional needs and

PART 3

Introduction

We are sick. As a society, America is very, very sick. If you have any doubts about how sick we are, look at how many medications are available to people without any prescription. How many medications are your friends and family taking? That number should be a wake-up call about the poor state of the health of Americans. If you are still in doubt, how many people do you know who struggle with cancer, heart disease, type 2 diabetes, depression, anxiety, infertility, or any other chronic diseases? One or two generations ago, those problems were virtually nonexistent. Now, they are becoming more the norm rather than the exception.

Medication is able to mask the symptoms of the diseases that we face. Statins can lower cholesterol but are unable to reverse heart disease or heal the body so that it is able to regulate its own cholesterol levels. Antidepressants can boost levels of serotonin, the "feel good" hormone, but are unable to heal the brain. In addition, medications come with a host of side effects that can cause other health problems, leading to a perceived need for more medication. The cause of these diseases is something that medication is unable to treat: poor diet. Aristotle, however, is credited with saying that food should be your medicine. The plant-based diet is a way to treat the cause of disease rather than medicating away the symptoms. It is just what America needs to regain its health.

Chapter 1: Obesity and the Standard American Diet

The Obesity Epidemic

There is no question that America is facing an obesity epidemic. An epidemic is a medical crisis that affects large parts of a population. With approximately eighty million adults and fifteen million children dealing with obesity, it has become one of the biggest health concerns today.

There is much more to obesity than being fat because obesity leads to many health problems. It is often correlated with high levels of blood sugar and insulin resistance, which, left unchecked, lead to type 2 diabetes. Excess fat in the abdominal area puts extra strain on the lumbar spine; in fact, just ten extra pounds of abdominal fat creates the equivalent of a hundred pounds of pressure on the spine. For this reason, obese people tend to suffer from back pain, sometimes to the extent that their daily routines and quality of life are affected. Extra fat places strain on the skeleton, leading many obese people to suffer from joint problems, particularly in the ankles, which bear most of the body's weight. The excess fat can build up in the blood vessels and visceral organs, leading to problems such as cardiovascular disease (including high blood pressure, heart attack, stroke, coronary artery disease, and congestive heart failure), respiratory difficulty, and fatty liver disease (which can mimic the effects of long-term alcohol abuse). Obesity can lead to hormonal disruptions, which can cause problems such as acne, polycystic ovary syndrome (PCOS) in women, and metabolic syndrome (a condition in which the body's ability to carry out its basic functions is compromised). Obese people are also more prone to sleep problems, such as sleep apnea, which occurs when the airway becomes partially blocked, causing the person to consistently wake up throughout the night. In addition to the physical problems, people who are obese also tend to struggle with emotional issues. These include challenges with self-esteem, body image, and social anxiety. Clearly, obesity is a problem that needs to be addressed and taken seriously.

While other components, such as genetics or metabolic disorders, may play a role in obesity, the main culprit leading to obesity is lifestyle choices, chiefly diet and exercise. In the nineteenth and early twentieth centuries, Americans were much more active because their lifestyles required it. People who worked on farms would be up milking cows, plowing fields, baling hay, planting crops, and harvesting from sunup to sundown. Think for a minute about how much physical energy farm work consumes! In the cities, most people did not have access to automated transportation, such as cars. Therefore, they mostly walked to their destinations, including work, school, and the grocery store. Furthermore, they did not have processed foods but only fruits, vegetables, grains, dairy, nuts, and meat that came from farms.

Today, many Americans have largely sedentary lifestyles. They drive to work, take the elevator instead of walking up the stairs, sit in chairs at their desks all day, drive home, and then watch television. Instead of bringing a healthy meal from home, many go out to eat for lunch, filling their diets with processed food and lots of sugar and little fiber (even if the food is labeled as healthy). With people getting little to no fiber, the sugar gets into the bloodstream, causing a sharp rise in insulin. High levels of insulin are linked to metabolic syndrome, weight gain, hormonal imbalances (insulin itself is a hormone), and diabetes. Instead of getting burned off through exercise, the sugar goes into the body's cells — usually much, much more than the cells require — and becomes converted into fat. Years of abusing the body through poor diet choices and lack of exercise lead to disease and a marked decrease in quality of life for individuals. As a society, it leads to a crippling burden on the medical system, causing resources (personnel, research dollars, lab equipment, etc.) that could be used to research and treat other conditions (such as pediatric cancer or spinal cord injuries) to be disproportionately allocated to treat the diseases associated with obesity.

Note that the text said "the diseases associated with obesity." The modern medical system is not as interested in treating obesity, the underlying cause of many of the diseases. The fact is that you cannot medicate yourself into health. A doctor cannot prescribe a pill that will make a patient healthy. The battle against obesity begins not in the doctor's office but in the kitchen, with the foods that people eat.

Why Are We so Fat?

The number one culprit behind the unprecedented weight gain of Americans is sugar. So many of the foods that we eat contain large amounts of added sugar; this is not only referring to sweets. Things as seemingly innocent as tomato soup and salad dressing are loaded with extra sugar. Americans consume far, far too much sugar.

The Problem with Calories

The problem with calories is essentially twofold. The first problem is that many people are not able to properly use the calories that they consume. Calories are necessary for the body to be able to function optimally. Calories are units of energy, so ideally, the number of calories that you consume will determine how much energy you have. However, the situation for many people is different, as their bodies lack the necessary vitamins and minerals needed to process that energy. That is why you may feel sluggish and tired after eating a large slice of cake (following the sugar rush, of course), which is high in calories but virtually devoid of nutrients.

The second problem with calories is that most Americans consume far, far too many of them. Not only are they not only able to properly use their calories, but the excessive number indirectly leads to weight gain. Notice that this said "indirectly" leads to weight gain, as calories themselves are not the culprit. Rather, the foods that contain the inordinate number of calories are to blame. Foods that are high in calories tend to be heavily processed and devoid of nutrients and come in supersized portions. For example, a hamburger found in a kid's happy meal is actually closer to how much an adult should consume; meanwhile, the kids eat the adult-sized hamburger while the adults eat the massive Big Mac and wash it down with a milkshake. Even processed foods that are low-calorie are deceptive, as they are also devoid of nutrients, largely unsatisfying (causing many people to consume far more than one serving), and can lead to weight gain. Nutritious foods, such as fresh fruits and vegetables, grass-fed beef, and free-range poultry are not only lower in calories than processed food but also much higher in nutrients, causing you to eat less. People who eat these foods feel full sooner, are more satisfied, and are all-around healthier.

The fact is that not all calories are created equal. One gram of sugar has four calories, while one gram of fat has nine calories. Simple arithmetic says to eat foods high in sugar rather than foods high in fat. However, this overly simplistic solution overlooks how our bodies actually use calories. Processed sugar is not necessary for the body to properly function; rather, it is hugely detrimental. In addition, if sugar is not immediately burned off, it quickly turns into fat. Furthermore, sugar has consistently been proven to actually increase someone's appetite, causing the person to consume far more than he or she normally would. While fat has more calories than sugar, there are some good types of fat that your body needs to be able to function properly. These include some saturated fats (found in free-range, grass-fed, organic animal products such as milk, beef, and eggs), omega-3 fatty acids (found in eggs and nuts), and monounsaturated fat (found in nuts and avocados). The body responds to these fats in vastly different ways than it responds to the lab-created fats — such as hydrogenated oils — found in processed foods. Eating good fats causes you to feel full, leading you to actually consume fewer calories while giving your body what it needs.

All of this is to say that instead of counting calories, what you really should be doing is paying more attention to the foods that contain those calories.

The American Diet

The typical American diet relies too much on convenience, so much so that people are willing to compromise their own physical health rather than be bothered with worrying about what they are eating. Breakfast food options in many supermarkets are centered on convenience rather than nutrition: sugary cereals, Pop-tarts, frozen breakfast sandwiches, and instant oatmeal. Most of these processed options have had most of their nutritional contents removed (instant oatmeal has far less fiber and other nutrients than steel-cut oats) and lots of sugar added. They are also devoid of fresh fruit (despite many of the claims on packages). Sadly, many people consume these products rather than making a nutritious breakfast that includes fresh fruit and protein. When office workers go out to lunch every day rather than bringing a healthy, pre-packed lunch from home, the reason is usually because going to a restaurant is more convenient than waking up fifteen minutes earlier. Going to a drive-through after a long day of work is so much more convenient than preparing a nutritious meal from scratch.

The result of all this convenience is way, way too many carbs, too much sodium, and too much unhealthy fat, such as hydrogenated oils, and far too few nutrients, such as vitamins, minerals, and fiber. Some people think that they can correct this imbalance by taking a multivitamin and fiber supplement every morning. However, the quality of the vitamins and minerals in supplements is of lower quality than of those found in fresh food, and they don't exist in the natural combination that our bodies require for optimal processing. In fact, the body only absorbs about ten to twenty percent of the nutrients found in a multivitamin. Fiber supplements can be of assistance, especially to people who are elderly but cannot produce all the benefits of including fiber in the diet throughout the day. Those benefits include lower levels of blood sugar and insulin and feeling full for longer.

What may be shocking to many people is that a lot of Americans are malnourished! This type of malnourishment is not the result of an inadequate amount of food but by poor food choices. Furthermore, excessive sugar actually reduces the body's ability to absorb the nutrients that it does receive. Many Americans have critically low levels of crucial vitamins such as D, K, and the B complex, which prohibit their bodies from being able to function optimally. This is yet another reason why so many people are sick.

Abdominal Fat Problem: Fastest Place to Lose Weight

One of the most dangerous places for the body to store fat is in the abdominal area; excess abdominal fat is so dangerous that it is actually a predictor of conditions such as heart disease and type 2 diabetes. The good news is that abdominal fat is the easiest type to lose. You don't have to do crunches or sit-ups to lose it; rather, you simply need to change your diet.

Abdominal fat is created by poor diet choices, such as excessive sugar, alcohol, and processed foods that contain unhealthy fats. In order to start losing it, eat foods that are low in sugar and other refined carbs, high in fiber, and high in protein. Examples include fresh fruits and vegetables, homemade soups and stews, and nuts and seeds. To further fight the belly bulge, rather than doing abdominal exercises, the best exercise to do is cardio, such as brisk walking and swimming.

Problems and Trappings of a High-Carb Diet

Americans consume far, far too much sugar and other refined carbs. Even though carbs are lower in calories than fats, they lead to weight gain. Refined carbs actually "flip a switch" inside the brain that signals that you need to keep eating more carbs. Furthermore, a few hours afterward, you may have a craving to eat more carbs. As a result, you end up consuming an excessive amount of empty calories instead of giving your body the nutrition that it needs.

In summary, Americans are facing an unprecedented health crisis brought on not by lack of food, but by an overabundance of food. Americans are consuming far too many calories, but are actually malnourished because the calories that they consume are not filled with the nutrients that they need for their bodies to function properly. Furthermore, too many Americans lack an understanding of what calories really are and what our bodies need in order to use them as energy. As a result, much of the population is fat and sick.

Chapter 2: Knowledge About Proper Nutrition

What Causes High Blood Sugar and High Blood Pressure?

High blood sugar exists when the bloodstream is filled with more sugar than it can process. When sugar enters the bloodstream, insulin is secreted by the pancreas to enable the body's cells to absorb the sugar and use it for energy. However, if there is more sugar in the bloodstream than the cells need, it builds up and insulin levels remain high. Over time, high insulin levels cause the cells to stop responding to it as efficiently, so more is required for them to absorb the sugar from the blood. If this is not corrected, the result can be insulin resistance. Insulin resistance will cause blood sugar levels to remain high, no matter how much insulin is secreted. If left untreated, diabetes can ensue.

The cause of high blood sugar is simple: too much sugar and not enough fiber in the diet. When sugar is consumed with fiber — for example, in fresh fruit, which contains sugar but also contains fiber — it released into the bloodstream more slowly, giving the body time to allow the cells to absorb it. However, when sugar is consumed without any fiber — for example, in a soda or piece of cake — it jets into the bloodstream, causing blood sugar levels to rise.

Blood pressure refers to the force of blood pressing against the walls of blood vessels; high blood pressure means that the blood is pressing too hard, which, over time, can cause damage to the cardiovascular system. The blood vessels can become stiff and hard, a sometimes fatal condition referred to as atherosclerosis. Poor diet choices are also behind many cases of high blood pressure. While there is a genetic component for *some* cases of high blood pressure, it is more often than not linked to the typical American diet. Rather than being linked to excessive sugar intake, high blood pressure seems to be more associated with excessive salt (most processed foods have very high levels of sodium) and bad fats, such as hydrogenated oils.

Lectins and Why They Are Bad

Lectins are proteins that bind to both cell membranes and sugar. They are found in nearly all plants and animals because they help cells communicate with each other. However, they can be very dangerous. One reason why is that some lectins are extremely toxic. For example, ricin, a toxin that is fatal in extremely small amounts, is derived from the lectins found in the castor bean.

Another reason why lectins are so dangerous is that they cause inflammation. Inflammation is one of the body's natural defenses against infection and other foreign invaders. However, over time, inflammation can lead to heart disease, hormonal disruptions, aches and pains, and a host of other problems. In addition, lectins can contribute to leaky gut syndrome, something that will be explained in detail in Chapter 7.

Lectins are found in nearly all of the foods that we consume. However, the biggest culprits include white potatoes, eggplant, beans, and dairy. Dairy poses a double danger because it is actually designed to penetrate the lining of the intestine, the cause of the leaky gut syndrome. These seemingly healthy foods should be avoided at all costs.

In summary, many Americans struggle with high blood sugar and high blood pressure. However, they do not understand how their poor diets and lifestyle choices are actually creating these problems. High blood sugar and high blood pressure are caused by consuming sugary processed food; high blood pressure is also the result of eating too much meat. These conditions can actually be reversed by changing eating patterns. In addition, lectins are proteins found in nearly all foods but are toxic, especially when consumed in large amounts. While plant-based foods should be consumed in favor of processed foods and meat, special care should be taken to avoid lectins.

Chapter 3: Lack of Exercise

Have you ever bought a gym membership at the beginning of the year? Gyms tend to heavily discount their memberships to entice the hordes of people making New Year's resolutions about getting fit and losing weight. They aren't taking a risk by offering their product/service at a rate that is too low because they know that within a month, most of the people who bought a membership will forget that they even have it. Most of those gym memberships will be used for a few weeks before being forgotten for the rest of the year.

This highlights the fact that Americans get far too little exercise. Our lifestyles have become quite sedentary, exemplified by the long hours that we sit at desks using computers (both at work and at home) and how much time we spend watching television. While for our ancestors' exercise was built into their daily routines, through activities such as hunting, farming, and walking long distances, we don't really need to exercise to get through the day. There are exceptions, such as occupations that require people to be on their feet constantly or those that involve heavy labor. However, for the most part, we are able to get through our lives just fine without any exercise. This lack of exercise is taking a huge toll on the nation's health. Not only are we consuming far too much sugar and processed foods, but we are not burning off any of those excessive calories.

The benefits of exercise beyond burning calories are tremendous. Exercise releases endorphins, which boost the mood; therefore, exercise is nature's own antidepressant. Chronic stress, something that many Americans struggle with (some without even realizing it, because stress has become such a normal part of life), causes hormones such as cortisol and adrenaline to be released into the bloodstream. High levels of cortisol are known to lead to weight gain, especially in the abdominal area. Exercise, however, burns off cortisol and other hormones that, over time, can cause damage. Exercise helps people sleep better at night, improves heart health, regulates and even decreases appetite, produces more mental clarity, lowers blood pressure, and burns off excessive blood sugar. With all of these benefits, in addition to burning calories, it is a wonder that exercise is not prescribed more than medication!

In summary, the benefits of exercise cannot be overstated. It increases bone and muscle strength, strengthens the heart, improves blood flow, and boosts mood. However, too many Americans lead largely sedentary lives that are practically devoid of exercise. As a result, their bodies are not able to function properly and they are chronically lethargic and fatigued. Instead of dealing with the root of the problem — lack of exercise — many opt for expensive and dangerous medications.

Chapter 4: Downfall of Medication

When is the last time you saw a commercial or online advertisement about lawsuits for people who took a certain medication and experienced dangerous side effects? When is the last time you saw a commercial or online advertisement for a particular medication, and in the fine print was a list of dozens of harmful side effects, some of which could be life-threatening? Up until 1985, advertising prescription medications directly to consumers rather than to doctors was illegal. However, nowadays our media is inundated with ads for prescription medications, and as a society, we have become fixated on the idea that a pill can cure most, if not all, of our ailments.

What Medication Does to Your Body

The reality is that while medication can alleviate some symptoms and be very beneficial in critical cases, it can also be very damaging to the body. This section will look at different types of medication and the harm that they can cause.

Antidepressants. Approximately 10% of the US population is on antidepressants, and they are the third most prescribed category of medication. Most antidepressants work by preventing neurons from reabsorbing the hormone serotonin, the "feel-good" hormone. This raises overall serotonin levels, but over time, causes an imbalance of serotonin inside and outside of neurons. Because serotonin does more than elevating mood (it also aids in the growth and death of neurons, digestion, reproduction, and blood clotting), imbalanced levels can lead to problems such as digestive problems (including abdominal bleeding), sexual dysfunction, and sleep disturbances. Furthermore, after prolonged use (even just a few months), the brain begins to push back after the effects of the drug in order to restore the proper balance of serotonin. This can lead to a full-blown relapse of depression, even while people are still taking the medication. Commonly, doctors will either increase the dose or switch patients to a stronger antidepressant without appreciating that the brain itself is working against the drug.

Painkillers. Painkillers are usually taken in the form of over-the-counter medication to alleviate discomfort associated with aches and pains, including menstrual cramps and arthritis. While many people are aware of the dangers of narcotic painkillers, even OTC ones are harmful. They work by preventing nerves from being able to carry out their functions, namely, to transmit messages from different parts of the body to the brain. Long-term use can actually lead to nerve damage. In addition, they are harmful to the liver and can cause stomach bleeding, which can be fatal.

Antibiotics. Antibiotics are commonly prescribed to treat bacterial infections, such as respiratory infections. They work by killing off the bacteria inside the body. However, the body naturally contains good bacteria, including approximately five pounds of it in the gut alone! This gut bacteria are known as the microbiome and are essential to carrying out many vital functions, including absorption of nutrients and regulation of hormones. Because antibiotics are indiscriminate in the bacteria that they kill, they devastate the microbiome and therefore disrupt many of the body's natural processes.

In addition, strains of bacteria are becoming resistant to antibiotics. This is because as a nation, we have become so dependent on medications, believing that a pill can fix all of our health problems, that we have overused antibiotics. Some patients are so insistent on getting medicated for whatever ailments they have that they are prescribed antibiotics for viruses, such as colds, something that antibiotics are powerless against. In response, the bacteria develop defenses to protect them from the antibiotics. The result is that new and difficult-to-treat diseases, such as MRSA, are becoming increasingly common.

Ultimately, medication is able to alleviate the symptoms of the disease, but it is not able to cure the overall dysfunction that led to the problem. Statins can lower cholesterol, but they cannot fix the cause of high cholesterol: poor diet and lack of exercise. Antibiotics can fight off foreign invaders that lead to infection, but they cannot heal the body so that it is able to defend itself through its natural mechanisms without antibiotics. If you want to actually address the cause of your symptoms rather than become a revolving-door patient, you need to fix and change your diet.

In summary, there is no benefit that medication can provide that adequate nutrition and exercise cannot provide, but without the damaging side effects. Exercise is more effective at treating depression and anxiety than antidepressants and other mood-enhancing medications. Having an optimized microbiome in the gut, fed with plenty of high-fiber fruits, vegetables, and probiotics, cannot only treat infections better than antibiotics but can eliminate the pathogens before they even take hold. Our lifestyles are what have made us sick, and medication cannot fix a lifestyle problem. Medications are dangerous and produce side effects that can pose long-term health risks. A healthy plant-based diet, however, can replace the need for medication.

Chapter 5: Case Studies of Places with the Highest Longevity

Despite its reputation for being wealthy and prosperous, the United States actually ranks number 50 in the world in terms of life expectancy, with Americans living an average of just over 78 years. Countries that fare better have several things in common, including social factors that cause people to lead healthier lifestyles. The world's highest life expectancy — nearly 90 years — is found in Monaco, which also has the world's highest population of millionaires and billionaires. Since most of the rest of us can't afford the kind of lifestyle that may contribute to the high longevity of residents of Monaco, that and other small, wealthy states will be disregarded.

Okinawa, Japan. The Japanese inhabitants of the island of Okinawa eat a low-fat diet that largely consists of fish, tofu, seaweed, and vegetables. Many of them actually only consume 1200 calories a day; however, their life expectancy is approximately 87 years, three years longer than their other Japanese compatriots. In fact, Okinawa has five times as many centenarians as the rest of Japan! Many Okinawans remain healthy until the end of their lives, and those who are 80 years old may have bodies that more closely resemble that of someone in his or her forties or fifties.

Loma Linda, California. Loma Linda is a small town of about 25,000 people, about sixty miles from Los Angeles. It is the center of the Seventh-Day Adventist Church, which advocates a plant-based diet and strongly discourages smoking. The different lifestyle habits of the church's members may be what contributes to the fact that its residents enjoy a life expectancy of about 85 years, as compared to the rest of the United States, which is only about 78 years.

Iceland. The small Nordic country of Iceland has an average life expectancy of just under 83 years, the highest in Europe. It also has exceptionally low infant mortality. These results can be at least partially attributed to the clean energy used to provide for the nation's power needs. However, they can also be attributed to the traditional diet of Iceland, which is high in fish, and a culture that promotes being physically active, especially outdoors.

In summary, cultures that promote the highest rates of longevity have several things in common. The people tend to be more active than in other parts of the world, thereby reaping the myriad benefits of exercise. Their diets are low in meat and other animal products and high in fruits and vegetables.

Chapter 6: Who This Book Is For

If you are struggling with any health problems, even those that may be genetic, then this book is for you. This chapter will look at what the plant-based diet can do for many common health problems.

Autoimmune disease. An autoimmune disease results when the body's immune system believes that healthy cells are foreign invaders and attacks them as such. Examples of autoimmune diseases include Crohn's, rheumatoid arthritis, and multiple sclerosis. Chronic inflammation is believed to be one of the causes; in fact, it is the culprit behind many chronic diseases. Inflammation is triggered by foods high in sugar and excessive consumption of meat, especially processed meat. Eating a diet mostly from plants results not only in less inflammation but a reversal of the damage caused by long-term inflammation! Many people with autoimmune diseases who have switched to a plant-based diet have noticed not only that their symptoms are largely alleviated but also that the disease itself becomes reversed.

Irritable bowel syndrome (IBS). IBS is a condition that affects as much as 15% of the American population; it results in intestinal dysfunction, including cramping, bloating, diarrhea, abdominal pain, gas, and constipation. Eating a plant-based diet has proven to considerably help people with IBS. Fresh fruits and vegetables are high in prebiotics, which promote a healthy environment for the good bacteria that make up the colon's microbiome. Proper functioning of the microbiome is essential to bowel health, as well as the health of the rest of the body.

Brain fog. Brain fog, or a generalized lack of clarity, can be substantially helped by eating a plant-based diet. When your body is out of whack, usually caused by poor diet choices and lack of exercise, your mood and thinking can be dramatically affected. Giving your body the nutrition that it needs will ameliorate most, if not all of the problems that are contributing to fuzzy and clouded thinking as well as a depressed mood.

Arthritis. Arthritis, a painful joint condition, is caused largely by chronic inflammation in the joints. As previously stated, inflammation is caused by eating a diet high in refined carbs, especially sugars, and meat, especially processed meat. However, a plant-based diet will not only bring down inflammation but can actually reduce the damage caused by long-term chronic inflammation.

High blood pressure. Eating a lot of salt, as part of a diet high in processed food and low in fruits and vegetables, is the primary contributing factor to high blood pressure. Studies have shown that reduced consumption of meat — consuming only one or two servings a week — resulted in most participants, blood pressure was reduced by about 25%. This result was achieved without a drug supplement. Going to a full vegetarian diet reduced blood pressure by up to 40%.

High cholesterol. Cholesterol is found exclusively in animal products. Plants on their own do not produce cholesterol. Our bodies naturally produce some cholesterol, which is generally considered to be of the beneficial type. However, high consumption of meat and products derived from animals, results in high levels of bad cholesterol, which can lead to heart disease and other problems. Switching to a plant-based diet will naturally lower your cholesterol levels simply because you won't be consuming nearly as much.

Heart disease. The reason that heart disease is the primary cause of death in America is because of poor diets and lack of exercise. Americans fill their days with sedentary activities and lots of processed, sugary foods that are also high in sodium. Eating much less meat, especially red meat, eliminating sugar and processed food, and eating mostly vegetable- and fruit-based foods have been shown to dramatically lower rates of heart disease and even reverse it in people who already suffer from it.

Acid reflux. Acid reflux is a condition in which stomach acid is propelled upwards into the esophagus, causing a burning sensation. While one out of five Americans suffers from acid reflux, in rural African villages, the risk was only one in one thousand, making it virtually unheard of. Most foods in the American diet are highly acidic, thereby contributing to the symptoms. However, plant-based foods are more alkaline, or basic, and bases neutralize acids.

Overweight or obese. People who are overweight or obese and switch to a plant-based diet, rather than relying on low-calorie processed foods, lose much more weight. Feeding your body what it needs, instead of what tastes better, results in feelings of fullness, satiation, and fewer calories consumed. Further, because those calories are useful and used efficiently by the body, people have more energy and are able to exercise more.

Those who want to look healthier. When people want to brighten their complexions, look younger, and generally look healthier, they usually go to a salon for an expensive treatment or buy a skin cream. While these procedures may make people look healthier, true health comes from the inside and is reflected in the outer appearance. In other words, when people are healthy on the inside, they look healthy on the outside.

Reverse aging. Processed foods loaded with chemicals and sugar, along with large amounts of meat and dairy, cause our bodies to age faster. However, a plant-based diet can actually reverse some of the signs and symptoms of aging. While it can't reverse the aging process, it can slow it down. Telomeres are structures at the end of our cells' DNA that keep the double-helix structure from unwinding. Every time a cell divides, the telomere is weakened, leading to the effects of aging. Telomerase is an enzyme that helps rebuild telomeres, and a plant-based diet is linked with stronger telomerase activity. What this means is that a plant-based diet can help reverse some of the effects of aging and even slow the aging process.

In summary, many of the diseases that plague modern society are the direct result of poor lifestyle choices. Changing the way that we eat can reverse and even eliminate not only short-term infections and other acute diseases but also chronic diseases, as well. All of this is to say that whoever you are, whatever health problems you may be struggling with, the plant-based miracle diet is for you.

Chapter 7: Leaky Gut Syndrome

What is Leaky Gut Syndrome?

Leaky gut syndrome, like obesity, is becoming a national epidemic due to poor foot choices by much of the American population. The leaky gut syndrome has also been called intestinal hyperpermeability. The walls of the intestine are porous so that the nutrients in food can be absorbed into the bloodstream. However, in leaky gut, they become excessively porous, to the point that larger portions of undigested food, including waste and toxins, to enter the bloodstream. In response, the body begins to attack the foreign invaders. The liver works hard to filter out all of the food macromolecules but is unable to keep up with their constant flow into the bloodstream. The immune system then kicks in and attacks the macromolecules. They are then absorbed into the body's tissues, resulting in inflammation. As you have already seen, chronic inflammation is at the root of many diseases. Instead of carrying out its normal functions, such as filtering the blood and reducing inflammation, your body will actually go to war against itself, which can result in autoimmune disease.

Fungus Theory

Candida is a fungus that can live in your intestines; one theory about the origin of leaky gut syndrome is that it is the result of an overgrowth of candida. The theory states when a candida yeast infection grows unchecked, the fungus grows "roots" into the walls of the intestines. The wall of the intestine becomes overly porous, allowing large particles of undigested food to pass into the bloodstream.

Plant Protein

Protein from some plant sources, such as soy and wheat (wheat protein is gluten), should be avoided at all costs, as they are considered to be "anti-nutrients." Celiac disease, or gluten intolerance, is related to the leaky gut syndrome in that consuming gluten can actually lead to a 70% increase in intestinal permeability. Soy protein is just as bad; not only is

90% of soy genetically modified (which leads to a host of other problems) but on a molecular level, it mimics gluten. As a result, soy protein can also dramatically increase intestinal permeability.

Intestinal Irritants

Intestinal irritants can be behind many cases of leaky gut syndrome. There is no universal list of intestinal irritants; rather, the foods that should be avoided are, to some extent, particular to the individual. However, some of the most common culprits are caffeine, wheat (specifically, the gluten found in wheat), sugar, and soy. When foods that are intestinal irritants to you enter the bowel, they can pass through the bowel membrane and into the bloodstream.

To find what foods are problematic for you, eliminate consumption of one item at a time, for two weeks, and then gradually reintroduce it back into your diet to see what effect it has. For example, eliminate all dairy products for two weeks. Keep a journal to gauge whether you feel better or worse. At the end of two weeks, gradually begin consuming dairy again. Do you feel better or worse? If you feel worse when consuming it, dairy is probably an intestinal irritant for you.

There may be other foods that are intestinal irritants for you that are not on the general list. If you are still having problems, you may need to see a specialist to determine exactly what foods should be avoided, at least until your gut heals.

Lectin Plant Proteins

Lectins are proteins found in nearly all foods; they are produced by plants and therefore consumed by animals that eat plants. Thus, they make their way into the entire food system. Consumption of lectins cannot be avoided; however, you should try to limit them as much as possible, especially if you are dealing with leaky gut syndrome.

Lectins are problematic for leaky gut syndrome because they gravitate towards areas like the lining of the gut, where they attach themselves and cause intestinal damage. Eliminating all grains and soy, which tend to be very high in lectins, will help heal your gut. Once the lining is restored, you can gradually add back in grains that have been fermented and sprouted; these grains have smaller amounts of lectins.

Whole Grains and Resistant Starches

Whole grains are usually described as healthy. However, that is only partially true, as they may be healthier than their refined (white) counterparts in areas such as glycemic index. In fact, whole grain bread is higher in lectins than white bread because the refining process significantly reduces the amount of lectins. Consider that the grains harvested to make bread and other foods are actually the seeds of plants. If all of a plant's seeds were eaten, that plant would become extinct; therefore, nature evolved a way to prevent seeds from being eaten. Seeds have a hard shell that is lined with lectins and other anti-nutrients, to keep them from being eaten. This reason is why whole grains, even more than white grains, contribute to leaky gut syndrome.

Instead of whole grains, opt for sprouted grains. Sprouted grains have been allowed to germinate before being milled into flour, thereby eliminating the toxins contained in the shell of the seed. Sprouted grains have significantly fewer lectins but still retain the nutrient content (unlike white, refined grains). Many kinds of bread now, such as Ezekiel bread, are being made from sprouted grains.

Potatoes and beans are often heralded as "resistant starches," meaning that the starch isn't digested and the calories are not absorbed. However, potatoes, beans, and other resistant starches are high in saponin, which actually creates holes in the cells that line the intestines. Even just a small amount of the cellular damage created by saponins can prevent nutrients from being transported by the cells. Furthermore, these resistant starches contain something called protease inhibitors, which increase levels of trypsin. Trypsin is an enzyme that damages the connections between the cells that line the intestines, thereby increasing the gut's permeability.

In summary, leaky gut syndrome is one of the diseases plaguing modern society because it is caused by poor diet. It is behind many cases of inflammation, abdominal discomfort, autoimmune disease, and toxins in the blood. Leaky gut syndrome is brought on by eating foods high in lectins, including seemingly healthy whole grains and beans. It is also caused by eating genetically modified food, dairy, caffeine, and any other foods that may be particularly irritating to you as an individual.

All of this may sound like a long list of foods to be avoided. However, the plant-based miracle diet is more about increasing your palate and enjoying foods that you would never have even considered.

Chapter 8: The Plant-Based Miracle Diet

What is the Plant-Based Miracle Diet?

Rather than being an eating plan that you stick to for a set period of time, the plant-based miracle diet is essentially a revolution of lifestyle in which permanent lifestyle changes are made. Instead of opting for eating a certain number of calories each day or getting into an exercise regimen until certain results are achieved, the plant-based miracle diet is about eliminating all processed foods eating only whole foods or those that are minimally processed.

There are three forms of the plant-based miracle diet; whichever one you decide will depend on your body type, goals, and the lifestyle changes that you are willing to make. The first form allows for some consumption of meat, as long as it is only free-range, grass-fed, and organic. Modern farming methods aim to raise animals as quickly as possible so as to create the most profit for the food company; therefore, animals raised for their meat are fed subpar food that includes unused body parts from other animals, plastic pellets, and even manure. The animals often live in unhealthy conditions, being crammed into cages that are too small and living on top of each other. They aren't able to get any exercise, and as a result of these conditions, the animals themselves are sick. To keep them from getting sick and to help them grow faster, many animals are fed a steady stream of antibiotics (most antibiotics used today are for farming). Consider that anytime you eat conventional meat, you are consuming a sick animal. That reason alone is enough to make the switch to eating only meat that is organic, grass-fed, and free range. However, the bulk of the diet consists of fruits and vegetables, and meat is eaten no more than two or three times a week.

The second form of this diet is vegetarianism, which includes the consumption of wild-caught fish (rather than farmed fish, which are subject to many of the farming methods listed above) and organic eggs from free-range chickens or other poultry. The third form of this diet is complete veganism, in which absolutely no animal products are consumed.

Choosing what works for you may be a process in which you make some lifestyle changes, such as eating more fruits and vegetables while reducing your consumption of meat until you switch to vegetarianism. You may be entirely unable or unwilling to make the switch to vegetarianism, but you make sure that all of your meat is from healthy animals rather than those raised in a factory farm. You may already be a vegetarian but want to incorporate more fruits and vegetables into your diet until you transition all the way to veganism. Whichever choice is best for you, make sure that the changes you make are ones that you can and will stick with.

In addition to a significantly reduced meat consumption, the plant-based miracle diet is, well, about eating more plant-based foods. Conventional wisdom, such as the food pyramid, says that we should aim to eat five servings of fruits and vegetables a day. This mindset sets us up for the belief that we should add fruits and vegetables into the diet that we already consume, thereby making it healthy. For example, when eating out you may decide to substitute a side salad for fries, thereby making your meal healthy. However, nothing could be further from the truth. The side salad might add one serving of vegetables to a meal loaded with hydrogenated oil, refined carbohydrates, sugar, and trans fat. It can hardly begin to offset the damaging effects of this meal.

The entire diet actually needs to be overhauled, not to make room for more fruits and vegetables, but to make plant-based foods the foundation on which the entire diet is built. Instead of ordering a side salad with a hamburger or slice of pizza, the salad should be the main dish of the meal, possibly with a small amount of meat added as a topping. Instead of eating a bowl of cereal that claims to have fruit added, the fruit should be the centerpiece of breakfast. A bowl of fruit with sprouted-grain toast and an egg would be a much healthier, plant-based option.

Because so much of the American diet is built around convenience, making the change to a plant-based diet is not just changing the foods you eat but changing your entire lifestyle. You have to change the way that you think about food. Food is not meant to be convenient or something that you eat mindlessly throughout the day. Rather, it is the source from which your body derives its health. Aristotle is credited with saying that food should be your medicine. That should be your attitude about food.

If you must have coffee in the morning, instead of stopping by Starbucks on the way to work or even filling up at the office coffee pot, make a pot of organic coffee at home (coffee has some of the highest levels of pesticides and other chemicals of any crop in the world). Instead of going out to lunch because it is easier than preparing a lunch at home, make the lifestyle changes necessary in order to either prepare your lunch the night before or wake up ten minutes earlier so that you can prepare it in the morning. Invest in a slow cooker so that healthy soups and stews can cook while you are at work, and a healthy plant-based supper will be waiting for you when you get home.

The way that you shop for groceries will have to change. If you are used to clipping coupons and buying foods that are on sale, you will have to completely change how you think about buying food. Some foods, such as conventional, factory-farm milk and wheat-based products, are subsidized by the US government to keep the prices low for consumers while still giving the farmers a profit. However, as you have seen, these foods contribute to many of the health problems that are plaguing Americans today. Instead of opting for foods that are cheap or convenient, such as microwavable frozen dinners, go first to the organic part of the produce section. By far, the bulk of what you buy should be in this section.

Other options for procuring plant-based foods include going local. Farmers markets are great places to find produce and grass-fed meat that is raised by small, local farmers. While conventional produce may be grown on the other side of the world and picked before it is ripe so that it can be shipped to the United States, the produce at a farmer's market is usually picked either that day or the day before. Because small farmers are not usually subsidized and their costs tend to be higher than those of conventional farmers, the foods found at farmer's markets can be more expensive. If you qualify for programs such as WIC, they can help offset the cost. The quality of the food and value to the local economy, rather than big agricultural corporations, make the higher cost worth it.

Besides a farmer's market, you can also see if there are any pick-your-own farms in your area. A pick-your-own farm grows the produce, but local people go in and pick it. You pay after you are finished picking; the cost is based on the weight of produce that you picked. The farmers don't weigh you before and after, so you are free to eat as much as you want while you are out picking! Going to a pick-your-own farm can be a great family outing in which children learn more about food and where it comes from while being able to procure it for themselves. It will certainly be a different type of outing than a trip to the movies or a favorite restaurant!

As you can probably see, the plant-based diet involves more than simply changing what you eat. It is changing how you think about food and, in turn, making lifestyle changes to accommodate the new mindset.

Why Should You Get on This Diet?

As previously explained, many, if not most, of the health problems facing Americans today are related directly to the foods that they eat. Refined carbohydrates, especially sugar, cause a slew of problems ranging from metabolic syndrome, weight gain, and obesity, destruction of the microbiome, to insulin resistance and diabetes. Some have been tricked into believing that they can make a healthy switch from refined carbs to whole grains, such as swapping out their white bread for whole wheat bread. However, while whole grains have a lower glycemic index than refined carbs, they are high in lectins, which can damage the wall of the intestines and lead to leaky gut syndrome. Lack of adequate vitamins and minerals due to not eating enough fruits and vegetables causes problems with immunity, blood clotting, and other disorders that are commonly associated with malnutrition.

So many of these problems can be fixed — and are getting fixed — by getting onto the plant-based diet. Eliminating all processed foods and eating only whole foods is proving across the board to have a marked effect on people's health and even curing diseases, such as diabetes and terminal cancer, that were believed to be irreversible. Furthermore, a plant-based diet leads to higher levels of energy and a better mood, leading to an overall higher quality of life.

How to Attain a Clean Diet

Most of the foods that are grown through conventional methods are "dirty." This means that not only are the methods used to grow them very destructive to the environment (large amounts of wasted water, water being contaminated by sewage, large amounts of energy needed to transport them), but they are also loaded with pesticides and other chemicals that are not safe for human consumption. Many of the pesticides that the FDA has labeled "safe" are far more dangerous to both humans and the environment than the DDT that was outlawed in 1972.

In addition to high levels of pesticides, some major biotechnical companies, such as Monsanto and Syngenta, have manufactured genetically modified seeds. GMOs are touted as having unique benefits because of the DNA that was changed, allowing them to have properties such as being resistant to drought, having higher levels of certain vitamins, or being able to withstand the stronger pesticides sprayed on them. GMOs are so ubiquitous today that unless the label on your food says that it is organic or non-GMO, you can be certain that it does contain GMOs. GMOs are very harmful to human health on two main fronts. The first is that they contain particularly high levels of the dangerous pesticide glyphosate, which is a known carcinogen. The second is that it actually changes the DNA of some human cells and the bacteria that make up the gut's microbiome. It should come as no surprise that the rise of GMOs and the rise of the leaky gut syndrome have happened simultaneously. Furthermore, GMOs are incredibly destructive to the environment and have the potential to permanently alter the DNA of some species.

Many of these chemicals are stored in the liver, which acts as a filter. However, when the liver becomes overloaded because so many chemicals are entering our bodies, the chemicals are stored in fat cells.

Because the body needs a place to store these toxins, it will refuse to get rid of excess fat cells. Losing weight can have as much to do with the chemicals in our food as with the food itself.

With this in mind, eating a plant-based diet is not enough. You need to ensure that the "healthy" whole foods that you are consuming are also clean, meaning free from these dangerous chemicals. The two ways to ensure that your food is not loaded with chemicals is to either make sure that it is labeled as GMO-free or organic or buy it locally from small farmers.

Scientific Mechanisms Behind the Plant-Based Diet

Genes are behind some of the diseases that we face. For example, some scientists have proposed that there is actually a genetic tendency for some people to gain weight easier and have a harder time losing it than other people. Some people are genetically more prone to addictive behaviors, such as smoking and overeating. Diseases such as cancer and Alzheimer's even have a genetic component! Genes are seen as an insurmountable obstacle to overcoming disease and attaining health and wellness. However, more and more studies are showing that a healthy lifestyle built around the plant-based diet can actually have more of an impact on disease, health, and well-being than genes.

In most cases, genes on their own do not cause disease (exceptions include childhood diseases such as cystic fibrosis). Rather, they predispose people to become more likely to develop a disease. For example, Mary Grace may have a gene that makes her more susceptible to developing breast cancer. All people have some number of cancerous cells in their bodies at all times, but they are usually destroyed by healthy cells that are properly functioning. Mary Grace's faulty gene may work in such a way that breast cells are more prone to turning into dangerous cancer cells, and the healthy remaining cells are less able to destroy the cancerous cells. That tendency can be either mitigated or augmented by her lifestyle. If she eats lots of damaging sugar and processed foods, her healthy cells will be even less capable of protecting her from cancerous cells. However, if she eats a diet that is based on organic, plant-based foods, she will be providing her healthy cells with the ability to fight off and destroy the cancerous cells. Furthermore, she will be giving the healthy cells the nutrients that they need to keep from mutating into cancerous cells in the first place. This example is just one way of how the plant-based miracle diet can override a person's genes and promote overall wellness.

In summary, the plant-based diet is a complete change of lifestyle, from one that is based on convenience and leads to disease, to one based on an understanding of health, well-being, and how certain foods contribute to an enhanced quality of life. It is not a list of foods that you can and can't eat, a point system, or measure of calories. You can't go to the grocery store and just buy a different brand of chips or cookies that are formulated to be compatible with this diet. Rather, you have to change how you think about food and be willing to make the necessary lifestyle changes to make whole, plant-based foods the centerpiece of your diet. These lifestyle changes include filling your shopping cart with produce rather than grains and meats, cooking meals at home (usually from scratch) instead of eating out, and eating food that is organic. The benefits produced by the plant-based diet — added years to life and life to years — make all of the effort worth it.

Chapter 9: Benefits of the Plant-Based Miracle Diet

Stabilize Blood Sugar and Blood Pressure

High blood sugar and high blood pressure are some of the biggest health woes causing disease today. However, the plant-based miracle diet can help stabilize and even reverse the conditions.

The elimination of all processed foods means that sugar consumption is drastically reduced; most sugars come from fruits and the breakdown of sprouted grains. As natural sources of sugar, these foods also contain high levels of fiber, which slows the sugar's absorption as well as the uptake of insulin. Because less sugar is entering the bloodstream, less insulin is needed to transport it to cells for energy. Even if someone already has developed insulin resistance, meaning that increasingly high levels of insulin are required to process the sugar, consuming less sugar means that less insulin will be required. Less sugar entering the blood, coupled with that sugar being processed efficiently by insulin so that it can be used by the cells, means that excess blood sugar is completely eradicated. Over time, stabilized blood sugar can lead to insulin resistance being reversed.

Sugar is a highly addictive substance, even more addictive than some illegal drugs. For the first few weeks, you may feel the effects of sugar withdrawal, which can include headaches, lightheadedness, anxiety, depression, moodiness, and irritability. You may be tempted to say that your blood sugar is too low and you need to eat a dessert to bring it back up. However, added sugars have absolutely no health benefit. Instead, you should eat fruit (a well-made fruit salad can satisfy a sweet tooth) and sprouted grains, which will keep your blood sugar stabilized instead of causing it to spike and then plummet.

In addition to helping stabilize your blood sugar, the plant-based miracle diet can help stabilize high blood pressure. The main culprits behind high blood pressure are obesity, which causes the heart to work harder, and processed food, which contains the bad fats, sugar, and salt that lead to heart disease. Eliminating processed foods can have almost immediate effects on blood pressure; a plant-based diet can lower it by up to 30% in weeks. Because a plant-based diet naturally leads to weight loss, it causes the heart to work less hard but more efficiently, thereby also lowering blood pressure.

Other Benefits

People who eat a plant-based diet have significantly lower rates of obesity; in fact, the plant-based miracle diet is the single most effective way of losing weight and keeping it off. As previously mentioned, obesity is linked to many health problems, including heart and cardiovascular disease, type 2 diabetes, metabolic syndrome, and high levels of stress. While in the 20th century and earlier most disease was due to starvation and malnourishment, obesity-related diseases are actually the product of a combination of overnutrition (too many calories) and malnutrition (not enough vitamins, minerals, and fiber).

When fiber intake is increased and the body is getting (and absorbing) enough nutrients, the excess weight begins to melt off. With reduced levels of sugar, hormones such as insulin become stabilized. Hormonal diseases, such as metabolic syndrome, insulin resistance, and type 2 diabetes, start to reverse. The wall of the gut begins to heal itself and the microbiome becomes healthy, causing problems such as autoimmune diseases and IBS to disappear without any medicinal intervention. The mood elevates, alleviating or even eliminating psychological problems such as depression and anxiety. Hardened arterial walls begin to soften, causing blood pressure to lower and thereby reducing the risk of stroke and other heart diseases. Without trans fats and bad cholesterol, arterial blockages are reduced and even eliminated, allowing for blood to flow freely throughout the body.

In summary, the benefits of the plant-based diet simply cannot be overstated. One of its most immediate effects is that high levels of blood sugar and high blood pressure begin to drop and reach safe, stable levels. In addition, it allows the body to heal itself so that other diseases and health problems, such as high cholesterol, obesity, and autoimmune diseases, are able to resolve themselves.

Chapter 10: Other Options and Diet

The Atkins Diet

The Atkins Diet took the United States by storm in the late 1990s and early 2000s. Dr. Robert C. Atkins promoted the diet and wrote a book about it in 1972. The theory behind it is that carbs are the reason we gain weight, so limiting carbs as much as possible leads to weight loss. People on the diet are advised to restrict consumption of any starchy or sugary foods, such as potatoes, bananas, wheat, apples, juice, and candy. The payoff is that they can eat as much protein (meat) and good fat as they want.

When Dr. Atkins began advocating this approach in the second half of the twentieth century, nutritionists and doctors were aghast. Fat was believed to be the enemy, and sugar was, for the most part, harmless (sugary processed foods like Snack Wells became popular during the 1980s and 1990s as diet foods). However, our understanding of nutrition has changed; we now understand that sugar is far worse, and fat in natural forms, such as olive oil and the fat in avocados, can actually be beneficial. Artificial fats, such as hydrogenated oils and trans fats, are to be avoided. Many people have boasted of being able to successfully lose weight on the Atkins diet. Proponents claim that it increases energy levels and actually reduces the risk of heart disease.

Unfortunately, the Atkins diet does not advocate exercise, claiming that it is not necessary for weight loss. Furthermore, the severely reduced consumption of carbs actually leads to eating fewer vegetables and almost no fruits, causing your body to not get the nutrients that it needs. Atkins is actually an animal-based diet.

The South Beach Diet

As the Atkins diet craze began to subside, the new South Beach diet began to rise in popularity. Its appeal over the Atkins diet was that it allowed for carbs to be incorporated. The push of the South Beach diet is the glycemic index, which determines whether particular carbs are good or bad. The glycemic index is a measure of how much and how quickly particular carbs will raise your blood sugar; whole grains are encouraged because they have a low glycemic index, while refined carbs and sugar are restricted because they have a high glycemic index. The South Beach diet promotes consumption of lean protein, whole grains, good fats, and fruits and vegetables.

One benefit of the South Beach diet is that it is more sustainable than the Atkins diet. The sheer amount of meat consumed on the Atkins diet is so high that on a global level, it is not environmentally sustainable. On a personal level, it can become very expensive, very quickly. Because the South Beach diet advocates a moderate intake of low-fat meat, such as chicken and fish, it is more environmentally and personally feasible. More people are able to follow it long-term because it allows for a moderate consumption of carbs. The higher intake of fruits and vegetables, over the Atkins diet, means that people on the South Beach diet are getting more nutrients. However, as you have previously read, the consumption of whole grains means more lectins, which lead to leaky gut syndrome.

The Paleo Diet

One of the latest diets to hit the US is the so-called paleo diet. The premise of the paleo diet is that our bodies evolved to process certain foods, the ones that our paleolithic ancestors ate. These foods included fruits and vegetables, lean meats, nuts and seeds, and fish. Modern farming began approximately 10,000 years ago; foods associated with modern farming are not compatible with the way that our bodies evolved. These foods include dairy, grains, and legumes. Modern processed foods and any added sugar are absolutely avoided.

The paleo diet has proven to be more beneficial than the Atkins or South Beach diets. Benefits of the paleo diet include decreased leptins, especially since grains and legumes are eliminated. It naturally includes a higher amount of fruits and vegetables to compensate for the lack of grains. Because our paleolithic ancestors were always active, the paleo diet advocates exercise every day; exercise has proven to be beneficial to both physical and emotional health. Even though the paleo diet is not a weight-loss formula, advocates say that they lose weight on it. They also have increased glucose tolerance, lower levels of triglycerides, and a stabilized appetite. However, the paleo diet does not address the problem of lectins.

Why the Plant-Based Diet is Best

The plant-based diet is the best of all of these other diet plans because, rather than being primarily a means to lose weight, it addresses the root causes of disease and advocates a healthy lifestyle. Reducing consumption of meat is shown to reduce blood pressure; eliminating it completely reduces it even more. In addition, raising animals for meat consumes far more environmental resources than growing the plants that underlie the plant-based diet. The plant-based diet addresses critical areas, such as the microbiome and lining of the intestines, that are ignored by even the paleo diet. The plant-based diet is better for humans and for the environment.

In summary, the plant-based diet is not a fad or a means for quick weight loss. While weight loss is a result, that is merely a side benefit. Its goal is overall health and well-being. In addition to being better for your own personal health, the plant-based diet is better for the environment.

Chapter 11: Myths and Dangers

The world of health food and diets has become so commercialized that any diet comes with a host of critics and advocates, and along with them, seemingly contradictory information. If you do a Google search for veganism, vegetarianism, Atkins diet, plant-based diet, lectins, or any number of terms associated with healthy eating, you will receive so many different accounts, based on different information, that you may be tempted to forego healthy eating altogether. Knowing what to feed our bodies for optimal health and well-being seems to be the insurmountable task. There are some myths associated with the plant-based miracle diet, which this chapter will explain and dispel. It will also highlight some of the dangers of a plant-based diet, with the purpose of giving you the information you need to overcome them.

Myth 1: Whole grains and dairy are important sources of vital nutrients.

Despite the growing prevalence of leaky gut syndrome and increasing evidence that it is correlated with, if not caused by, dairy and the lectins found in whole grains, many nutritionists insist that both are necessary components of a healthy diet because of the nutrients found in them. However, there are no nutrients found in whole grains and dairy that can't be found elsewhere. Green, leafy vegetables, such as broccoli, kale, spinach, and parsley, are high in the B vitamins commonly found in whole grains but without the high level of lectins, as well as the calcium touted by dairy. Consuming these foods will not only reduce the amount of lectin you ingest and therefore help heal your intestinal lining but will also increase the prebiotics that feed your gut's microbiome.

Myth 2: Animal protein is superior to plant protein.

Other primates, including gorillas, have muscles that are far bigger than ours. However, they derive virtually all of their protein from plant sources. The fact is that amino acids are created by plants, which are then consumed by animals. Animals create some amino acids, but these can be obtained from plants. In fact, all plants contain all nine essential amino acids; therefore, consuming a sufficient amount of plant-based food will ensure that you get enough protein. The rule of thumb is that if you are getting enough calories from a plant-based diet, then you are getting enough protein.

Myth 3: A plant-based diet is prohibitively expensive.

Healthier food is certainly more expensive, especially when placed side-by-side with its processed counterparts. If a loaf of white bread costs one dollar and a loaf of sprouted-grain bread costs five dollars, one can easily conclude that healthy food is five times more expensive. However, that is only part of the actual situation.

Most Americans go out to eat between three and five times per week. If the average cost of a restaurant meal is ten dollars, then that is as much as fifty dollars a week going to unhealthy restaurant food! If you put that much money towards buying plant-based food rather than convenient restaurant food, you will probably end up spending about the same amount.

Many people on a plant-based diet report that they actually spend less on food than they previously did when eating a diet high in animal products and grains. Furthermore, they spend less on health-related issues, making the savings even more.

Myth 4: B12 is only found in meat.

Vitamin B12 is actually created by bacteria, not by animals. Animal products contain B12 because the bacteria in the animals create the B12. Properly fermented vegetable-based foods, such as natto (fermented soy), can be used to meet a person's B12 needs.

Danger 1: Plants don't contain Vitamin A in the form that our bodies need.

Our bodies need Vitamin A in the form of retinol, but what plants give us is beta-carotene, which is then converted into retinol. Based on conditions such as the health of your gut, your thyroid function, and some genetic factors, your body's ability to convert beta-carotene into retinol could be compromised. In order to avoid this danger, take the necessary steps to ensure that your gut is properly functioning so that it can properly convert beta-carotene into retinol. You may want to get a periodic blood test to ensure that you have appropriate levels of Vitamin A.

Danger 2: Not consuming animal products can reduce the amount of stomach acid, thereby reducing the overall efficiency of the digestive system.

When you consume animal products, especially meat, your stomach creates more hydrochloric acid (stomach acid) to assist in the breakdown of proteins. The digestive process is driven largely by a balanced pH, meaning that stomach acid is necessary to kick-start digestion. Without adequate stomach acid, the body is actually less able to absorb the nutrients that you consume. This condition is called hypochlorhydria. It results in abdominal discomfort, bloating, and gas immediately after eating and can lead to malnutrition from lack of nutrient absorption.

In order to prevent hypochlorhydria, drink a cup of room-temperature water with a tablespoon of apple cider vinegar before meals. The apple cider vinegar will help stimulate the stomach to produce the necessary acid.

Also, keep in mind that digestion is not merely a physical process. It is actually a parasympathetic process that involves both the mind and the body. Emotional distress can actually impede digestion. Maintaining a stress-free lifestyle and being relaxed when you eat can also combat hypochlorhydria.

In summary, many of the reasons why people decide not to follow the plant-based diet are based on faulty logic and science. There are no nutrients found in animal sources that cannot also be derived from plants, and usually with higher quality. While there are potential dangers in following the plant-based diet, they can be alleviated by taking simple measures.

Chapter 12: The Importance of Nutrition

Even though Dr. Atkins claimed that exercise is not necessary for weight loss, it is a necessary aspect of overall health and well-being. Eighty percent of wellness is based on diet, while the other twenty percent is based on exercise. This chapter will look at that concept in more detail.

Eighty Percent Diet

It goes without saying that the food you eat is incredibly important. Proper nutrition can prevent many of the diseases associated with modern society and reverse them in people who already have them. This section will look at some important vitamins and minerals and give you information on what they do and what plant-based foods contain them.

Iron is a mineral usually obtained from red meat, but it is also present in green leafy vegetables, such as kale, spinach, and broccoli, as well as eggs and shellfish. It is required by red blood cells in order for them to transport oxygen throughout the body. Iron deficiency is known as anemia; it causes cells throughout the body to become hypoxic (lacking in oxygen). As a result, someone with anemia will feel weak, fatigued, and may even faint.

Vitamin D has gained a lot of popularity in the health community over the past few years, and for good reason. Its functions include allowing the body to absorb calcium, which is necessary for bone health, regulating the immune system so that it functions properly, and protecting against cancer. Low levels of vitamin D are linked with many different cancers, weight gain, heart disease, and depression. It can be obtained from egg yolks and wild fish, but the body actually produces it naturally from sunlight. In order to have optimum levels of vitamin D, the best thing to do is get plenty of sunshine.

Vitamin K is an unsung hero, as vitamin D has attracted so much attention. Vitamin K allows the blood to clot and aids in the transportation of calcium throughout the body, making it essential for healing injuries and protecting bone health. Without vitamin K, a simple wound can lead to so much blood flow that the injured person can resemble a hemophiliac. This important nutrient can be found in pretty much any fruit or vegetable that is green: Brussels sprouts, spinach, kiwi, avocado, broccoli, cabbage, kale, chard, and grapes.

Vitamin B1, or thiamine, is required by the body in order to process carbohydrates and proteins. Many people rely on whole grains to obtain thiamine, but it can also be found in nuts and some vegetables, such as peas.

Vitamin B2, or riboflavin, aids in the production of red blood cells and converting food into energy. Without an adequate supply of B2, no matter how many calories you consume, you will still feel lethargic. It can be obtained by eating almonds and asparagus and is also found in dark chicken meat.

Vitamin B6 is crucial because, like B2, it helps convert food into energy; it also aids in the breakdown of sugar, making it particularly beneficial for people who have developed insulin resistance or type 2 diabetes. It can be found in peas, spinach, and bananas; those who choose to consume small amounts of animal products can also find it in light poultry meat and eggs.

Vitamin C is touted for its ability to help boost people's immune systems. More than that, it is critical for the formation of collagen (the main protein found in the connective tissue between cells) and in creating some of the chemical messengers that the brain uses to transport its electrical signals. Sugary processed foods, such as gummy fruit snacks, and sugary juices like to boast of containing high levels of vitamin C; however, more than ample amounts of it can be found in nearly any fruit. Instead of drinking a glass of orange juice to help fight off a cold, eat a whole orange. You will get plenty of vitamin C that has not been subjected to the processing required to make orange juice; the whole orange will also provide you with the fiber needed to prevent a spike in blood sugar.

Vitamin E is a powerful antioxidant that protects cells from damage that can be incurred from toxins and the normal aging process. It is also important for skin health; medical professionals may apply pure vitamin E directly to a severe skin injury. It can be found in plant-based foods that are high in fat, such as olive oil, avocados, and nuts. Keep in mind that while some oils, such as corn, soy, canola, and vegetable oil, are also derived from plants, they are created in laboratories and are full of damaging trans fats. They should be avoided as often as possible.

Folate is particularly important for pregnant women because it helps prevent birth defects. It also aids in heart health and in the creation of red blood cells. Many people rely on grains, beans, and lentils to obtain it, but it can be found in plentiful supply in dark green vegetables.

Calcium is important for healthy bone growth and development, as well as for transporting messages between cells and helping muscles work. Its benefits are widely touted as part of a campaign to get Americans to drink more milk; however, milk contributes to leaky gut syndrome. Furthermore, the calcium found in milk is not the best kind. The best calcium can be found in broccoli and dark leafy vegetables. For those who opt to consume animal products, it is also found in fish and fish bones (which are edible).

Magnesium is another unsung hero in the arsenal of vitamins and minerals. It improves nerve function, decreases anxiety, improves sleep, alleviates muscle pain, improves heart health, prevents migraines, and relieves constipation. This vital mineral can be found in dark leafy greens, nuts, avocados, and bananas. It can also be obtained by taking a bath with Epsom salt.

Zinc helps boost immune function so that you can heal faster. It strengthens the hair, skin, and nails, and a plentiful supply of zinc can even diminish scars! Many Americans obtain zinc through red meat and poultry, but it can also be found in nuts and seafood. Zinc supplements can also be beneficial but are no substitute for a good diet.

Twenty Percent Exercise

If twenty percent of health and well-being is dependent on exercise, then without it, even the most nutritious diet in the world will only bring eighty percent of your health potential. The twenty-percent deficit could leave you prone to depression, anxiety, and physiological disease. This section will look at different types of exercise and the benefits that they can produce.

Cardio exercise is basically any exercise that raises the heart rate. It includes brisk walking, running, swimming, stair stepping, bike riding, rowing, and dancing, amongst other things. Cardio exercise produces many benefits, beginning with promoting heart health. Muscles are healthier when they are used, and the heart is no exception. Elevating the heart rate during 30-minute to hour-and-a-half sessions of cardio workouts can strengthen the heart so that it actually creates more capillaries, thereby allowing blood to flow more freely throughout the body. It also burns off unwelcome substances that can build up in the blood and other parts of the body, such as triglycerides, excess sugar, and stress hormones. As a result, it leads to weight loss, increased energy, elevated mood, and decreased stress. Whatever your exercise routine may be, you should make time for at least thirty minutes of cardio most days of the week.

Strength exercises help to keep your bones and muscles strong. They include lifting weights and resistance training, such as using resistance bands or resistance machines. Strength exercise is not just for the young; older people in particular benefit from it because it helps them maintain their independence and prevent falls.

Flexibility exercises help maintain a wide range of motion while keeping your body limber. The range of motion refers to the extent to which you are able to move different parts of your body; people with conditions such as bursitis can benefit from flexibility exercises, as they can help extend the range of motion and thereby help the person get back his or her abilities. Flexibility exercises include doing yoga and stretching various parts of the body.

Balance exercises, such as tai chi, standing on one foot, some yoga positions, and heel-to-toe walking, help to strengthen the body's core. A stronger core promotes overall health, especially digestive and gut health, and decreases the risk of diseases that begin in the abdomen (such as type 2 diabetes and some autoimmune diseases).

In summary, the plant-based diet is able to provide you with all of the nutrients necessary to achieve optimal functioning of the entire body. Even nutrients typically obtained from meat, such as iron.

Chapter 13: Safety, Side Effects, and Warnings

Despite its superior benefits, the plant-based miracle diet does not come without some of its vices. These vices, however, do not outweigh the benefits of the diet.

Many Americans are incredibly deficient in fiber; while 97% of Americans get enough protein (because of all the meat that they consume), 97% of Americans do not get enough fiber. The average fiber intake is only fifteen grams per day, while the body needs 32 grams per day! Switching to a plant-based diet means a significantly higher intake of fiber, which may take some adjusting. Common side effects of increased fiber intake include bloating, abdominal cramps, gas, and diarrhea. Less common side effects include temporary weight gain (usually from water) and constipation. In order to mitigate these side effects, make the switch to the plant-based diet gradually. Instead of immediately jumping from one or two servings of fruits and vegetables per day to ten, build that number up over the course of a few weeks. Not only will this allow your system to adjust, but it will also give you time to adjust your lifestyle to accommodate the plant-based diet.

One benefit of the plant-based diet is that it cleanses toxins that have accumulated in your body from years of unhealthy eating. Some people immediately feel great. However, for some people, this purge can lead to symptoms of detox, including aches and pains, fatigue, irritability, and other ailments commonly associated with the flu. Most Americans are addicted to sugar; sugar has actually hijacked their brains similar to narcotics and other addictive substances so that the brain is tricked into thinking that it has to have it. Switching to the plant-based diet may involve a withdrawal process, which can include anxiety, depression, intense cravings, moodiness, and brain fog. In order to mitigate these side effects, eat fruit whenever a sugar craving hits. Drinking a calming beverage, such as lemon balm tea, throughout the day can help lessen the anxiety and moodiness.

Consider the transition process, in which your body adjusts to the plant-based diet, as any transition process. Transitions are not ever easy. Think of it like getting a new puppy. The new puppy is cute, playful, and cuddly, so much so that you would not dream of getting rid of it. However, that puppy has to be house trained so as to not constantly do its business on the floor (or any other unwelcome place). This process involves completely changing your routine so that you are available every few hours to take the puppy outside. Furthermore, the puppy wants to chew on everything, including your expensive shoes. You have to learn to put all of your things away so that the puppy cannot chew on them, and will still have to replace some things that were important. However, as your routine adjusts to life with a puppy, you grow fond of it as it contributes to increasing your own happiness and quality of life. You love playing with it, and seeing it happy makes you happy. One day, you will look back on those days of adjustment to life with a puppy with fondness and won't even think about all the potty accidents or chewed-up shoes.

Likewise, when you make the transition to a plant-based diet, the process may be hard and require some serious adjusting. However, once your body gets used to it, you will feel so good and will have such an increased quality of life that you won't have any desire to go back.

Some people wonder whether the plant-based diet is for them. Simply put, the plant-based diet is for everyone. People of all ages and at all stages of life can benefit from it. Pregnant women who plan their meals appropriately can benefit immensely from the plant-based diet. It can counteract some of the fatigue and morning sickness brought on by pregnancy while still providing the developing baby with all of the nutrients necessary to thrive. In addition, pregnant women on the plant-based diet have a markedly lower chance of developing gestational diabetes and other pregnancy complications.

Children, even infants, can benefit from the plant-based diet. While infants need high levels of fat, this can be obtained from the mother's breast milk. Following the World Health Organization guidelines of breastfeeding for two years will ensure that your child will get all of the fat needed throughout the infant and toddler years. Children raised on the plant-based diet have fewer behavioral problems, including ADD and ADHD.

Athletes and bodybuilders are notorious for consuming large quantities of meat and other animal products in order to fuel their muscles for intense training sessions. However, they can get all of the nutrients that they need on a plant-based diet, especially one that calls for eating free-range, grass-fed meat once or twice a week. All of the nutrients needed for cellular and muscular growth and repair can be found in plants; small amounts of meat and other animal products can work as a supplement.

In summary, there are some drawbacks to the plant-based diet, but nothing that cannot be overcome. The uncomfortable effects of a drastic increase in fiber intake can be mitigated by gradually increasing the amount of fiber in the diet until optimal levels are achieved. The symptoms of detox that come from flushing the toxins from the body can be very uncomfortable, but again, a gradual transition can ease this process. Withdrawal from sugar addiction can be the hardest part of the transition for some people; to help get through it, eat a lot of fruit and drink herbal tea.

Chapter 14: The Light Dieters

Light dieters are individuals who want the benefits of the plant-based diet but are unable to make a commitment for a total change. They change one meal a day and aim to make the other two meals as healthy as possible. This chapter is specifically for people whose lifestyles may be inflexible due to occupational, financial, or any other reasons. Construction workers, athletes, shift workers, and others who need a lot of energy and are not able to take the time to deal with the side effects of going entirely plant-based are ideal candidates. People who want to experiment with the plant-based diet to see if it is something they can stick with are also ideal candidates. This regimen also applies to people who want to change to eating entirely a plant-based diet but are making the change gradually.

Changing One Meal a Day

Changing one meal a day from being meat-based to being plant-based is one way to substantially benefit your own health as well as the health of the planet. If every American switched one meal a week from being meat-based to being entirely vegan, the environmental equivalent would be like taking half a million cars off the road! To further increase the benefit both to your own health, the local economy, and the global environment make that one meal per day locally sourced from small farmers in your area.

The immediate benefits of changing one meal a day to being plant-based include that your daily servings of fruits and vegetables will go up. Many people rely on meat for their protein intake; however, some fruits and vegetables, such as jackfruit, are also high in protein as well as other vital vitamins and minerals. Choosing to use these plant-based sources of protein, even only one time each day, will provide the added benefit of extra fiber and other essential nutrients.

Your palate will expand as you try new fruits and vegetables that you previously had not even heard of. You may find that there are a lot of plant-based foods out there that you enjoy more than you did processed foods! This will encourage you to further increase your intake of a variety of fruits and vegetables and completely eliminate all processed foods. You may not even be tempted to go back to your old ways of eating.

Changing just one meal a day will allow you to gain many of the benefits of the plant-based diet, including improved overall health and vitality; reduction, reversal, and even elimination of chronic as well as acute diseases; and more energy. Furthermore, some of the unpleasant side effects — such as gas, bloating, diarrhea, and constipation — will be alleviated compared to those who make the full switch immediately. In other words, by changing just one meal a day to being completely plant-based, you should expect to feel better!

There is an important caveat, one known as the law of compensatory consumption. When we make positive changes, we tend to subconsciously justify doing more of our negative, detrimental habits because we feel so good about ourselves. For example, when people decide to use less water to help reduce their environmental footprints, they oftentimes subconsciously use more energy than they did previously; this is because they feel that their decreased water consumption justifies an increased use of electricity. People who switch to one plant-based meal a day will feel the temptation to eat more meat and processed foods at other meals. Be aware of this temptation so that you can resist it! Keep at the forefront of your mind the reason why you are making the switch to one plant-based meal per day so that you don't even want to eat more meat or processed foods. Don't fall prey to the law of compensatory consumption!

In summary, making the switch to eating one plant-based meal per day is a great way to kick off a lifestyle of healthy eating. You can begin to reap the benefits of the plant-based miracle diet but without many of the unpleasant side effects that can come with it. In addition, by making the change gradually, you are more likely to stick with the diet rather than if you jumped in all the way without giving yourself a transition period.

Chapter 15: Intermediate Dieters

Intermediate dieters are people who change two meals per day from being meat-based to being plant-based. Maybe they have already gone through the transition of changing one meal a day and can't get enough of the positive benefits. They want to continue making the switch to being entirely plant-based eaters. Other people who are ideal candidates for being intermediate dieters are those who have active social lives that include eating out with friends and/or family on a frequent basis. While restaurant meals almost inevitably contain animal products unless the menu says otherwise, eating a plant-based diet for two meals a day can compensate for the restaurant meals. In addition, busy moms whose families are resistant to eating a plant-based diet are ideal for changing two meals per day; they can eat a plant-based breakfast and lunch and then enjoy the same supper as their families. Meanwhile, all of the people making the switch to changing two meals a day from being meat-based to being plant-based are reaping even more of the rewards of the plant-based miracle diet.

Benefits, Expectations, and Results

The benefits of changing two meals per day from being meat-based to being plant-based are substantial. Most energy consumption in the sector of agriculture and food production comes from meat; it actually takes up to five times more water and a hundred times more food to produce a pound of meat as opposed to a pound of vegetables. The first benefit is a significantly reduced environmental impact. If the two plant-based meals that you eat each day are sourced from local small farmers and are organic (many small farmers use organic growing techniques, even if their produce is not certified as organic), the environmental impact is reduced even further. The second benefit is even more energy. While changing one meal a day to a plant-based diet increases energy levels substantially, changing two meals a day increases them even more. By giving your body the proper vitamins and minerals, as opposed to just the calories, that it needs, it is able to use the calories that it has consumed as energy. With that increased energy, you will *want* to exercise; rather than being a chore, exercise will become an indispensable part of your daily routine. Reaping all of the benefits of exercise is reason enough to make the change! Another benefit is increased alertness and improved mood. Brain fog, irritability, depression, and anxiety can all be caused, at least to an extent, by a poor diet that is high in processed foods and animal products. Eliminating processed foods and significantly reducing the number of animal products consumed can quickly turn those conditions around without any medication.

Just like with the one-meal-per-day switch, if you make the two-meal-per-day switch, you should expect to feel better. Your body will cleanse out more of the toxins that accumulated due to years of poor diet. While at first, you may experience some fatigue and withdrawal, especially if you didn't first make the transition to one plant-based meal per day, those effects are the result of your body being purged of all those toxins. After a few days, once your body has been cleansed, you will feel drastically better. Inflammation, and all of the problems that come with it — such as chronic aches and pains — will go down. Your gut will begin to heal, and its microbiome will be restored to optimal levels. In addition, excess weight will begin to fall off.

As with making the switch to one plant-based meal per day, make sure that you don't succumb to the law of compensatory consumption. Don't eat extra junk food to make up for all of the healthy food that you are now eating. If you must, splurge in another area. Get yourself a nice haircut or buy a new outfit to complement your now-healthy body. But don't steer off course! Then again, why would you even want to?

In summary, making the switch to eating two plant-based meals per day augments the benefits of eating one plant-based meal per day. Energy, vitality, and overall health and well-being are increased. The body flushes out the toxins that have accumulated and begins to heal itself, without the need for medication. The result is a happier and healthier you!

Chapter 16: Hard-Core Dieters

Hard-core dieting, in reference to the plant-based diet, is not an exercise in restriction or deprivation. Rather, it is a lifestyle of eating exclusively plant-based foods and reaping the benefits. While changing one or two meals a day is an ideal way for a lot of people to regain their health, especially people who are unwilling or unable to commit to an exclusively plant-based diet, going entirely vegan is for those who are completely committed to their health and well-being.

There are many lifestyle changes involved in eating nothing but the plant-based miracle diet. One of them is that socializing with friends will no longer involve going out to eat at any restaurant you or your friends should choose. Either the restaurant will have to have vegan options, or you will have to content yourself with watching everybody else eat. An alternative will be to invite friends over to your house for a vegan meal before going out on the town (or whatever you enjoy doing with your friends). An even better alternative is to not go solo when switching to the plant-based diet. See if any of your friends or family want to join in your endeavors. If no one wants to, at least try to earn the support of the people closest to you. That way, when you speak up about wanting to go to a restaurant that has vegan options, the people around you are more likely to acquiesce. They may even want to try vegan options, too!

Other lifestyle changes that you will probably encounter in the transition to full veganism include having to read food labels to determine if something is truly vegan and incorporating plant-based protein sources that aren't high in damaging lectins, such as natto. You will probably face some challenges in the transition, including the side effects mentioned in an earlier chapter. However, the benefits are life-changing.

People who went completely vegan for a mere 60 days reported that no matter how much they ate, they still lost weight. They experienced less soreness and had so much energy that they didn't know what to do with themselves. Six weeks in, they were prepared to make the transition permanent.

In summary, making the change to complete veganism is hard. It involves a lot of lifestyle changes and learning to eat in an entirely different way. However, it also leads to a revitalized body with exceptionally high energy levels.

Chapter 17: Going Organic

Dangers of Pesticide Use and Conventional Farming

In the year 1962, an American writer named Rachel Carson published a book entitled *Silent Spring*. The book highlighted how the use of heavy pesticides, including the supposedly safe one known as DDT, which was used commercially for agriculture and at home. The pesticide was known to cause cancer, yet was being sprayed indiscriminately into the environment. No long-term study had shown what its long-term environmental impact would be, but the bird population — including the emblematic bald eagle — was deteriorating because of its use. The title, *Silent Spring*, hearkened to the idea that with continued use of pesticides, we might experience a spring in which no birds sing. A public outcry ensued, which led to the banning of DDT in the year 1972.

Modern agricultural chemicals, however, may actually be worse than DDT. Glyphosate, the active ingredient in the commercially available pesticide Round-Up, was approved for use in 1974, shortly after the banning of DDT. Most bacteria are actually beneficial, especially those that comprise your gut's microbiome. Glyphosate actually kills most of the beneficial bacteria, both in the soil and in your gut. As a result, disease-causing bacteria are able to proliferate. It also damages the nutrients in the soil so that the plants are not able to properly absorb them, leading to sick plants and nutrient-deficient food. Glyphosate decreases the body's ability to detoxify foreign invaders and process organic compounds, further contributing to disease. Furthermore, it is toxic to human DNA, thereby holding the potential to devastate the entire human genome. It also disrupts the reproductive system, leading to problems such as infertility and birth defects.

Glyphosate has been linked with the rise of many diseases. For example, the rise in the use of glyphosate corresponds almost perfectly with the rise in autism spectrum disorder in children. It is a known carcinogen, meaning that it causes cancer, and may also be linked to Alzheimer's.

The environmental impact of glyphosate is unprecedented. It has built up in soils, damaging local micro-ecosystems. In fact, it has penetrated so deeply into the soil that it is contaminating water in the underground water table. Rainfall naturally causes glyphosate to runoff into streams and rivers, where it wreaks havoc on marine life. Fish are showing genetic abnormalities. Male fish are showing female characteristics, and some are even dying out. From rivers and streams, glyphosate makes its way into the ocean, where it continues its path of destruction. While Monsanto, the company that manufactures glyphosate, claims that it disintegrates rapidly, its residues can be detected in water two weeks to well over a month after exposure. In soil, it can be detected six months or longer after exposure.

Glyphosate is not even the worst chemical used commercially today. 2,4-D is the active ingredient herbicide found in many weed killers that can be bought at a store. Commercial farmers and local households use it to kill weeds. However, 2,4-D comprised about half of the chemical known as Agent Orange, which was sprayed indiscriminately in the jungles of Vietnam to help soldiers navigate them during the war. Agent Orange caused diseases in approximately one-quarter of the people exposed to it, including birth defects, genetic mutations, and cancer. The chemical that you may be using to spray your own yard to kill weeds may be one of the two ingredients that composed Agent Orange!

GMOs

In 1994, the Flavr Savr tomato, the first genetically modified food, was approved for commercial distribution and sale. Since then, GMOs, or genetically modified organisms, have proliferated to such a degree that unless explicitly labeled otherwise, you can be almost certain that what you are eating was genetically modified. Not only are plants genetically modified, but some animals are, as well. In fact, the first documented case of successful genetic modification was a mouse, in 1973. Today, genetically modified salmon are sold at supermarkets across the country. Genetically modified fish, known as GloFish and adored for their vibrant colors, are sold as pets. Genetically modified mosquitoes have been released into the wild to combat malaria and other mosquito-borne diseases.

Genetic modification is usually done to create some purported benefit. For example, some bananas have been genetically modified to help increase the body's ability to process vitamin A, and other crops have been genetically modified to make them drought resistant. The process of genetic modification involves isolating a particular desired gene, such as one that enables a crop to survive with less water, and inserting it into the genome of the candidate plant's seeds. This artificial manipulation creates plants that actually don't exist in nature. In addition, the benefit that the GMO plant is supposed to bring just doesn't come. Supposedly drought-resistant GMO crops are not able to withstand water shortages; in fact, they tend to do poorer than their non-GMO counterparts.

Eighty percent of GMO crops around the world are genetically modified to be resistant to herbicides and pesticides, especially the dangerous pesticide glyphosate. In fact, the company that creates most GMO seeds, Monsanto, is the same company that produces Round-Up! Crops that are genetically modified to withstand high levels of glyphosate are termed "Roundup Ready," and are specifically cultivated to be sprayed with glyphosate. Estimates are that approximately 300 million pounds of Roundup are sprayed every year globally. With the known and documented effects of Roundup on both human and environmental health, one can only shudder at what its extensive use is doing. In response, the weeds that Round-Up is supposed to be killing, while preserving the crop plants, are actually developing resistance to the herbicide, meaning that higher and higher levels of it are required.

GMO food poses a double threat to humans. The first is that the altered DNA actually changes the DNA of the bacteria in the microbiome, making them unable to perform their functions, and even changes the DNA in some of your body's cells. It is actually disrupting the human genome! The second is that it is loaded with glyphosate, exposing you to higher and higher levels of this toxic chemical. That apple that you think is a healthy snack, unless labeled as being organic or non-GMO, could actually cause infertility, cancer, hormonal disruptions, and genetic mutations!

Benefits of Organic Farming Techniques

As opposed to conventional, large agriculture, which relies heavily on the use of agrichemicals and leads to problems such as soil degradation and wasted water, organic farming uses techniques that are beneficial to the environment. Instead of artificial fertilizers, organic farming uses natural fertilizers, such as manure and compost. Instead of dangerous chemicals, it uses pesticides that are naturally created by plants or even insects, such as ladybugs. To keep the soil fertile, crop rotation is used. Instead of working against the environment by using artificial means to grow crops, it works with the environment by utilizing natural forces to produce a chemical-free crop.

Benefits of Eating Organic Food

The benefits of eating organic food over conventionally grown food are tremendous. People who switch to organic food routinely find that problems such as food allergies completely disappear. This could be because modern farming techniques, especially the cultivation of genetically modified food, is creating food sensitivities and allergies in otherwise healthy people. Another benefit is that people who eat organic food have substantially lower levels of chemical residue in their bodies. Therefore, they experience fewer of the health problems associated with high herbicide and pesticide use. In addition, because chemical toxins are often stored in fat cells, reducing those toxins can actually allow you to lose weight without necessarily reducing calorie intake! Because organic food is grown in healthier soil that retains its nutrients, it can even have a higher nutrient content than its conventional counterpart. All in all, organic food is better for you and for the environment.

In summary, modern, conventional farming techniques are devastating the health of the human population and of the planet. Heavy chemical use is damaging entire ecosystems, and GMO foods are causing even more extensive damage. However, organic farming techniques and the consumption of organic food hold great potential for reversing both environmental and human health problems.

Chapter 18: Complement to a Healthier You

The Ketogenic Diet

Our long-ago ancestors did not eat three meals a day, like we do. They hunted and foraged for food, and if there was no food, they simply didn't eat. However, in most cases, they didn't starve. Rather, their bodies adapted to this lifestyle by burning off fat as a primary energy source rather than sugar. In modern society, sugar is the most-used energy source, so much so that traditional nutritional wisdom says that glucose (a type of sugar) is the body's primary energy source. This reinforces the false idea that we need to eat a lot of carbs. Our bodies are actually very capable of using fat as a primary energy source; in fact, from a metabolic perspective, fat is a more stable and sustainable form of energy than sugar.

Ketones are substances created by the liver when it breaks down fat, thereby creating energy. Ketones are also important for brain health and mental function, so getting the body to create more ketones improves both the mind and body. The diet actually was developed as a way of treating neurological disorders! Most of the time, our bodies primarily rely on glucose, a simple form of sugar derived from carbs, as energy. As a result, the fat that is stored in our bodies is not burned; therefore, we are unable to lose weight. The ketogenic diet is about significantly reducing the amount of carbs eaten so that the body begins to burn fat liver produces the ketones to generate energy. Starving the body of carbs forces it into a metabolic state known as ketosis, which literally means that ketones are being broken down.

On the ketogenic diet, carbs only account for five to ten percent of all calories consumed, and those carbs come exclusively from fruits and vegetables. Seventy-five percent of all calories come from fat, and the remaining ones come from protein. The high-fat content is crucial to establishing an optimal state of ketosis; a high-fat diet also decreases hunger and appetite, as well as cravings for carbs. The fats should come from healthy, natural sources, such as avocados, unprocessed cheese, nuts, eggs, and red meat. The protein is derived from these high-fat foods. Variations on the ketogenic diet include cycling, with five days on and two days of high-carb intake, higher protein intake (suitable for athletes and bodybuilders), and adding in carbs around your workout schedule.

Because the body's own fat stores are being used for energy, the ketogenic diet quickly leads to weight loss. In addition, it has many other benefits, as well. The extremely low intake of carbs leads to greater mental clarity and performance, leading to increased productivity. Without insulin being generated to aid in the transportation of glucose, people on the ketogenic diet become more energetic and have a more regulated sense of being hungry and full. Lower, stabilized insulin can reverse the effects of insulin resistance and even type 2 diabetes. People with acne tend to benefit from the ketogenic diet as well, as it helps lead to clearer skin. Despite the high amount of fats consumed, it actually lowers cholesterol and blood pressure. In addition, the ketogenic diet has been the primary method of treating children with epilepsy for over a hundred years. It reduces the amount of medication that they have to take and leads to better outcomes. The ketogenic diet is also believed to reduce the risk, symptoms, and progression of Alzheimer's disease and aid in recovery from brain trauma.

The ketogenic diet has been shown to improve insulin levels in people who are diabetic and prediabetic, thereby alleviating the symptoms and even the disease. However, people who are diabetic should only go on the ketogenic diet under a doctor's supervision. Inability to create insulin means that glucose is unable to enter the cells to be used as energy, so the liver burns fats to create higher and higher levels of ketones. This can lead to a condition called ketoacidosis, which causes the body's pH to become so acidic that it can be fatal. Someone who does not have diabetes is at an immeasurably low risk of developing ketoacidosis; it usually only occurs in individuals whose diabetes is unmanaged.

Intermittent Fasting

Intermittent fasting is the process of starving the body of all calories so that it is forced into a metabolic state in which body fat is quickly burned and muscle is easily built. The idea behind it is that what you eat is not as important as when you eat; therefore, you don't have to give up any of the foods that you enjoy. Instead, you should only eat at certain times.

When food is consumed, the body spends about five hours digesting it; during digestion, hormones that lead to weight gain, especially insulin, are activated. Because most people eat within five hours of their last meal or snack, they are unable to enter into the stage in which they can lose weight because the fat-storing, weight-gaining hormones are constantly coursing through them. Intentionally foregoing meals by going through periods of fasting and feeding put the body into a state in which body fat is burned. You can drink as much water and calorie-free beverages (such as green tea and coffee) as you want but only eat at certain times. Fasting times usually range from 12 to 20 hours, but some programs have fasting periods that last as long as 36 hours.

The idea of intermittent fasting goes against traditional nutritional advice, which says that in order to keep the metabolism moving, you need to eat small meals all throughout the day. Eating small meals leads to a higher metabolic rate, while foregoing food puts the body into starvation mode, causing the metabolism to slow down and fat to be stockpiled. The problem with this traditional wisdom is that it is built on the idea that glucose, rather than fat, should be the body's primary energy source. In order for the body to continually provide energy through glucose, there does need to be a constant supply of food. However, that glucose raises insulin levels, leading to weight gain, not weight loss. The wisdom of intermittent fasting is that it relies on lowering insulin levels so that the body burns fat with little effort.

There are several different intermittent fasting programs, including LeanGains, the Warrior Diet, Fat Loss Forever, the Alternate Day Diet, and Eat Stop Eat. The Warrior Diet was one of the first diets to bring in the idea of intermittent fasting. It is based on the concept that in ancient civilizations (and even sometimes in modern ones), warriors or soldiers did not stop during the day to eat. Rather, they marched, trained, and battled during the day and only ate in the evenings. However, they were fit, alert, and capable of facing the enemy. On the Warrior Diet, you fast for 20 hours every day and consume all of your daily nutritional needs within a four-hour feeding window in the evenings. This regimen can be difficult to adopt all at once, so people on the Warrior Diet usually transition into it gradually. LeanGains is an intermittent fasting plan that incorporates workouts into the fasting and feeding schedule so as to optimize fat burn and muscle build. Other intermittent fasting plans, such as Fat Loss Forever and the Alternate Day Diet, use various schedules of feeding, fasting, and workouts so as to get the best results.

The benefits of intermittent fasting go beyond weight loss; it also helps improve cardiovascular health, energy levels, and mental clarity. Adjusting to intermittent fasting can be challenging, especially because until the body fully adjusts, periods of fasting can involve intense hunger, irritability, anxiety, and moodiness. Given time, the body is usually able to adjust quite well so as to reap the benefits of intermittent fasting. Some religious groups already advocate intermittent fasting, such as Muslims who fast during Ramadan. If fasting is already a part of your spiritual life, then intermittent fasting can be a way to kill two birds with one stone; you can get both the physical and spiritual benefits.

Many people can benefit from intermittent fasting. Those who have been trying to lose those last five or ten pounds, people who enjoy working out frequently, and people who already fast for reasons other than weight loss can benefit from implementing an intermittent fasting regimen. Pregnant women and people with certain diseases, including diabetes and ones that require a ketogenic diet (as opposed to being on a ketogenic diet voluntarily), should not try intermittent fasting. Additionally, some people have difficult schedules that can make intermittent fasting difficult, if not impossible. College students, shift workers, and people who must be on-call for work may have a very difficult time adapting an intermittent fasting program into their lifestyles. They may want to try another health and wellness program, such as the plant-based miracle diet or the ketogenic diet.

For more information, you can check out my book on intermittent fasting.

Exercise

The benefits of exercise are well-known and documented. People who exercise regularly experience lower levels of disease, higher levels of energy, a more moderated appetite, and higher overall health and well-being. Many people have been able to get off of a variety of medicines, everything from antidepressants to statins, because exercise alone was enough to alleviate the symptoms and even cure the underlying cause of illness. In order to get the most out of exercise, you need to get your heart rate above normal. While adding casual walks into your daily routine is beneficial in many ways, vigorous exercise that gets the heart pumping and forces you to breathe harder is the best. A brisk morning walk, taking the stairs at work, and a trip to the gym are all great ways to add heart-healthy exercise into your daily regimen.

Accountability Partners

Accountability partners are an important component of staying on track as you make the lifestyle changes necessary to become healthier. Your accountability partner may be someone who is more of a mentor that has already gone through the process; this mentorship set-up has shown to have great results in programs like Alcoholics Anonymous. Your accountability partner may also be a friend or peer who, like you, wants to get healthy. People who have accountability partners are much more successful at reaching their overall goals.

The key to having an effective accountability partnership is easy: Stay accountable to each other! Plan to connect with each other at least once a week to share how that week has been going. Did you fall off the wagon and into the sugar trap? Did you have a meat craving that you just couldn't ignore? How does your accountability partner deal with cravings? What are some of the benefits that you are seeing from your lifestyle changes? An accountability partner can give you an extra layer of vision that you don't have on your own because he or she can see things that you cannot. For example, you may see that the numbers on the scale haven't budged, but your accountability partner may notice that you look slimmer and your skin is brighter. He or she can also give you tips on other lifestyle changes that you can work into your daily or weekly routine.

Staying Motivated

Staying motivated while on a healthy eating lifestyle can be challenging sometimes, especially when you hit a weight-loss plateau (in which you are no longer able to lose weight) or when the holidays come around. Having an accountability partner and focusing on all the benefits that you are already seeing from your healthy eating lifestyle can help you stay on track. But what about in the beginning, when your whole body is sore from the toxins being purged from it and you don't think you will survive another sugar craving?

One necessary component of staying motivated is to make one change at a time rather than jumping in headfirst. Each time you make a change, be sure to replace the original with something even better. That way, you are easing yourself into a positive transition in which you actually like the replacement better; the changes will be much longer lasting than if you focus on deprivation and what you can't have. First, focus on eliminating sugar from your diet. Are you a heavy soda drinker? Start there. Throw out all the soda and get rid of all the excuses for needing it. No, you don't need to raise your blood sugar with a soda and no, you don't need the caffeine in it. Find a sugar-free alternative (not diet soda or anything that contains artificial sweeteners!). Kombucha is a fermented tea that still has a fizzy, slightly sweet taste but, unlike soda, has health-boosting probiotics, vitamins, and minerals. Many people have found that kombucha is a great alternative to soda. While it can be expensive to purchase (one bottle usually costs around three dollars), you can learn to make it at home for pennies a gallon.

Once the soda habit is gone, move on to your next sugar vice. Is it ice cream? A mid-afternoon crash that you solve with something sweet? Donuts? Find a suitable replacement for those things; instead of ice cream, use frozen bananas to make a smooth and creamy frozen snack. Eat frozen grapes; they can be a great way to satisfy a sweet tooth. For the mid-afternoon crash, plan ahead with a fruit salad that you will eat instead of going to the vending machine. Not only will you satisfy the need for something sweet, but you will have given your body an infusion of vitamins and minerals.

After a while, the gradual changes will start to snowball into a major lifestyle overhaul. Without you even thinking about it, that one vegan meal a day will become two. You'll want to take the stairs instead of the elevator because you love the feeling of getting the blood flowing. Give yourself enough choices, and you won't even miss the things that you thought you couldn't live without.

Habit Formation

Habits take between two weeks and one month to form. During the time when a habit is being formed, one slip-up can derail the entire process. The trick to forming a habit is to be aware of that fact so that you are equipped to not let those inevitable slip-ups get you completely off-track. Maybe you planned to go to the gym every Tuesday, Thursday, and Saturday. This Saturday, though, you just couldn't bring yourself to do it. Instead, you watched Netflix and ate grilled cheese sandwiches and drank soda. Before the end of the first season that you are binging on, you have convinced yourself that this healthy-eating lifestyle isn't for you and you can't do it, anyway. All of the efforts that you put into creating the necessary habits to enforce your lifestyle changes could easily be derailed at that point unless you are already aware of that potential.

The good news is that everybody has slip-ups. Everybody has bad days. And the best news is that that's perfectly OK! So, you had pizza delivered and ate four slices while going through two seasons of Game of Thrones instead of going to the gym. That does not make you a failure. It just means that you need to get up and start again tomorrow. Be kind to yourself, let yourself have a bad day, and then get back on track.

One key to preventing those slip-ups from becoming a regular occurrence is to try to figure out what causes them. Are you an emotional eater? Maybe a particularly stressful event or just feeling overwhelmed, rather than your own lack of willpower, led to you downing a pint of ice cream. Keep a journal so that you can stay on track of what keeps you motivated (what enables you to stay strong on good days) and what leads to you having a splurge.

Thirty days of healthy eating and regular exercise is usually enough to enforce the new lifestyle. However, remember that the most long-lasting changes are those that come gradually, so if you aren't able to become an immediate vegan and stay on track for 30 days, it's probably because you're trying to do too much at once. Get off of sugar for 30 days, and you will find that you no longer even want sweets. Then get off all processed food for 30 days, and you will find that you only want food that is fresh and nutritious. Next, exercise regularly for 30 days. You will find that you want to do it every day! Congratulations. You just developed the necessary habits to stay on track.

Foods to Focus on

One key to staying on track is to keep your eyes on the foods that you can focus on; there are far more foods that you can eat to support a healthy diet and lifestyle than foods that can derail it. Focus on continually expanding your palate to include more of the great variety of natural, plant-based foods that can help lead to overall health and well-being. Focus on eating plant-based foods that are grown without agrichemicals, to ensure that those toxins don't end up inside your body.

Fiber is a nutrient that passes through the digestive system unaltered; however, it slows the absorption of sugar and keeps you feeling full longer. Foods that are high in fiber should be consumed consistently. This does not include processed foods that have fiber artificially added to them, like Metamucil crackers or fiber powder. Rather, it refers to foods that are naturally high in fiber. Vegetables that are particularly high in fiber include celery, carrots, artichokes, Brussels sprouts, and broccoli. Fruits that are high in fiber include berries (raspberries, blackberries, strawberries, and blueberries), avocados, apples, oranges, and pears. The best part about eating fiber-rich fruit is that even though it is sweet enough to satisfy a sugar craving, the fiber in it keeps your blood sugar and insulin levels from spiking. To ensure that the fiber isn't destroyed, try to eat fruits and vegetables uncooked as much as possible.

Other foods that should be focused on are foods that are bright and colorful. While sweet potatoes are technically starches rather than vegetables, they have a nutrient profile that can rival most vegetables, while having a sweetness that can make them even more satisfying than white potatoes. Spirulina and chlorella are algae that are loaded with B vitamins; they make a great addition to smoothies. Turmeric is a bright yellow-orange seasoning that has health benefits so strong that it is superior to many medications! Experiment by using as many natural herbs and seasonings in your cooking as you can.

Work on continually expanding your palate to include more colorful fruits and vegetables. When you are first trying new ones, start by adding them to smoothies, soups, or salads so that you can adjust to the taste. You will find that there are plenty of foods that your taste buds are just waiting to discover and enjoy!

Foods to Avoid

On any healthy-eating plan, the first group of foods that should absolutely be avoided is anything that causes a spike in insulin levels. High insulin levels are behind many cases of obesity and disease, so keeping your insulin stable is necessary to getting your health back. Sugar, juice, white bread, soda, and pasta are just a few examples of insulin-spiking foods that should be avoided at all costs.

Lectins are substances found in plant proteins that can contribute to leaky gut syndrome, a condition in which the lining of the intestines becomes porous, allowing undigested food and toxins directly into the body. Virtually all foods contain lectins, so they cannot be completely avoided. However, some foods contain very high levels of lectins and should not be consumed. Beans and pulses, including kidney beans, navy beans, fava beans, lima beans, pinto beans, soybeans, mung beans, peas, and lentils are all high in lectins. Cooking destroys some of them, but not all. Grains and cereals, especially whole grains (because most of the lectins are found in the shell of the seed), are particularly high in lectins. These foods include barley, wheat, corn, rice, and wheat germ.

Genetically modified organisms (GMO food) should be avoided like the plague. Genetic modification alters the genome of an organism so that it is essentially a new breed that is not recognized in nature. The altered DNA can actually alter the DNA in your body's cells! In addition, GMOs are heavily sprayed with glyphosate, an herbicide that is known to cause cancer, hormonal disruptions, infertility, and a host of other health problems. In addition to the dangers GMOs pose to human health, they literally have the potential to completely destroy the planet. They inhibit biodiversity, which is crucial to healthy ecosystems. The glyphosate used to treat them has penetrated the water table, heavily contaminated the soil, and is wreaking havoc on marine and another animal life.

Supplements

Before considering taking supplements, remember that most of your nutritional needs should be met from the food that you eat. Supplements should be used only to enhance the nutritional benefits of food or to take the place of foods that you are unable to eat (for example, vegans often need to take supplements for the B complex). Use supplements in their most whole, natural form rather than chemically based supplements. For example, if you must use protein powder, use a brand that does not include chemicals in the powder and derives the protein from natural, rather than artificial, sources. Spirulina, chlorella, hemp, and chia seeds all make great supplements because they are entirely natural, come from plant-based sources, and can be added to food to make it more nutritious.

Some supplements can actually work adversely together to create a toxic brew in your blood. Talk to a doctor or pharmacist to ensure that any combination of supplements that you are taking is healthy.

BONUS

Introduction

Every vitamin and nutrient humans need can be found in a plant-based diet... including B12 and protein... Yes, protein. There are countless clinical studies that show a person does not need meat or even cheese in our diet. Not only will your body thank you, but Mother Earth would be appreciative if it could be personified.

One-third of all freshwater is used for livestock, and almost one-third of ice-free land on earth is used to grow grains and produce that is not used to feed human beings directly. This is a large amount of resources going to livestock which is used to feed the Earth's inhabitants. In this book, you will learn about plant-based eating, how it differs from veganism, and how plant-based eating can change your health for the better. This book will also touch base on a few scientific studies backing the decision to go animal-free... as well as an explanation of vitamin B12, vitamin D, iron, and protein.

The consumption of dairy, eggs, and meat can cause a myriad of health problems, and you will learn how you can get all your daily nutrition without eating a typical American diet. Included will also be a 30-day meal plan just in case you were not sure where to start. Eating a plant-based diet was considered radical many years ago, and even though you are amongst a select few who choose plants over meat...your numbers are growing and hopefully will continue.

Chapter One:

What is Plant-Based Eating? How Does It Differ From Veganism? What are The Health Benefits of Eating Plant-Based Food?

When people hear the words, "plant-based eating," they usually assume they would need to sacrifice good food for healthy living... this is not the case. Not only do you feel great when you make the switch, but you will find the food to be delicious and quite filling. Being plant-based is not about just eating salad. Salad will be very boring... probably after the second one. There is not a single person on earth who will like salad that much. There are so many different varieties of foods to eat, you just need to be creative, and sort of learn how to cook. So, what is a plant-based diet, you ask? This is a diet that consists of the consumption of whole grains, fruits, vegetables, nuts, legumes, and beans. You will eat a lot of different varieties of rice and potatoes if you are not concerned about carb-intake.

Which brings me to discuss the difference between veganism and a plant-based diet: Veganism is defined as the rejection of all animal products and animal by-products to further prevent the exploitation and suffering of animals. It is a lifestyle that is not just a diet, it includes the rejection of clothing, shoe, household product, and make-up companies that profit or participate in the maltreatment of animal. The products they purchase are frequently stamped with an encircled "V" with the sub-title "cruelty-free" underneath it. This differs greatly from simply being plant-based... this lifestyle is not usually based on the welfare of animals.

Plant-based lifestyle usually pertains to a healthy lifestyle that includes being active and only eating foods that originate from plants. Even though "veganism" and "plant-based" are often interchangeable terms and most people do not know the difference. A plant-based eater is specifically concerned for their health and how they can better it.

The benefits of going plant-based range from a healthy, glowing complexion to reducing the risk of developing cancer. According to Dr. David Katz, a practicing physician, and researcher at Yale Universities Prevention and Research Center, "A diet of minimally processed foods close to nature, predominantly plants, is decisively associated with health promotion and disease prevention." Plant-based diets are a surefire way to make sure you get all your vitamins and nutrients. If you plan your meals out properly and are willing to try the same foods in a new way, there's no reason why you should be vitamin-deficient (DISCLAIMER: This is not including chronic health problem where you have difficulties absorbing certain vitamins)

When you try to consume more wholesome foods like fruits, vegetables, whole grains, other complex carbohydrates, beans, legumes, nuts, seeds, and lots of water, you are allowing yourself fewer health problems. You are more likely to lose unnecessary weight, and you will have a significantly lower risk of heart disease. Eating less meat will reduce your risk of stroke, cardiovascular problems, and diabetes. Your blood pressure will be more regulated due to regular consumption of whole grains, Omega fatty acids, potassium, and less intake of sodium.

You will be able to manage your blood sugar by regularly consuming foods high in fiber. Fiber slows down the absorption of sugars in your bloodstream and keeps you full longer. Fiber-dense foods balance out your cortisol levels, which in turn will make you less stressed out. Also, when you switch to plant-based food, you will reduce your risk of developing cancer, like breast or colon. Inflammation may also subside; if you have arthritis, studies show that when you cut out dairy and meat from your diet, your arthritic symptoms can improve and reduce flare-ups. There are almost too many benefits to count, and way too many to list. The only way to see the broad spectrum of these benefits is to see for yourself.

Chapter Two:

Clinical Studies: Science-Backed Proof

A 2011 study[123] from Canada found 62.1% of Canadians to be overweight and 25.4% of the population to be obese. This study found vegans and vegetarians, regardless of gender, age, or location, to make up less than 6% of the obese/overweight population. Did you know that dietary cholesterol only comes from meat, fish, eggs, and milk? The same study found vegans to have significantly lower levels of cholesterol in their blood... which means a plant-based diet will not put you at risk to have clogged arteries or heart disease. Type 2 diabetes and cancer are both prevalent diseases of people

---

[1] Public Health Agency of Canada [website] Obesity in Canada: prevalence among adults. Ottawa, ON: Public Health Agency of Canada; 2011. Available from: www.phac-aspc.gc.ca/hp-ps/hl-mvs/oic-oac/adult-eng.php. Accessed 2018 May 14.
From <https://www.ncbi.nlm.nih.gov/pmc/articles/PMC5638464/>

[2] Statistics Canada [website] Body mass index of Canadian children and youth, 2009 to 2011. Ottawa, ON: Statistics Canada; 2013. Available from: www.statcan.gc.ca/pub/82-625-x/2012001/article/11712-eng.htm. Accessed 2018 May 12
From <https://www.ncbi.nlm.nih.gov/pmc/articles/PMC5638464/>

[3] Statistics Canada [website] Body composition of Canadian adults, 2009 to 2011. Ottawa, ON: Statistics Canada; 2013. Available from: www.statcan.gc.ca/pub/82-625-x/2012001/article/11708-eng.htm. Accessed 2018 May 12.
From <https://www.ncbi.nlm.nih.gov/pmc/articles/PMC5638464/>

who regularly consume animal products.

In 2015, the World Health Organization (W. H. O.) found evidence[4] linking red and processed meat consumption to colorectal cancer. This study has also found overwhelming evidence to classify processed meats such as sausages, bacon, ham, beef jerky, corned beef, smoked, fermented, and cured meats, as a group 1 carcinogen. The Academy of Nutrition and Dietetics stated that a vegan diet (when properly planned) could provide the prevention and treatment of many diseases and ailments-- it can be perfect for any person in any stage of life, including pregnancy, infancy, and athletic.

Aside from how animal products affect our health, maintenance of livestock has quite a negative impact on the Earth as well. The consumption of animal products uses an astonishing and disturbing amount of earthly resources. 60 Billion animals, per annum, are used to feed the human population. Livestock production is responsible for 18 % of the greenhouse

---

[4] World Health Organization [website] Carcinogenicity of consumption of red processed meat Lancet. Oncol. 2015 Dec; 16(16):1599-600.

gas emissions. That is more than all the vehicles on earth emit into the ozone layer. To produce a kilogram (2.2 pounds) of beef, it requires seventy times the amount of land required to produce the same amount of weight in vegetables. The amount of all irrigation water[5], the amount that is used to produce livestock is calculated to increase from 15% to 50% by 2025.

Another study[6] on people with rheumatoid arthritis, published in the journal of the American Dietetic Association in 2010, stated that when you switch to a plant-based diet, you will reduce your joint inflammation. There were significant improvements in joint tenderness, duration of stiffness in the morning, and better grip strength. Vitamins B-12 and D, Calcium, and Essential Fatty-Acids are essential for bone health. Fatty Acids are commonly found in olive and canola oils, chia, flax, and hemp seeds.

A study[7] from Massachusetts General Hospital associates high consumption levels of animal protein in the human diet with higher mortality rates. The longest study of the effects of different sources of

---

[5] A global assessment of the water footprint of farm animal products. 2012;15(3): 401-15. Epub 2012 Jan 24.

[6] A study done on vegan and vegetarian diets about joint health, *Journal of the American Dietetic Association, 2010.*
From < https://www.arthritis.org/living-with-arthritis/arthritis-diet/anti-inflammatory/vegan-and-vegetarian-diets.php>

[7] Edward Giovannucci et al. **Association of Animal and Plant Protein Intake With All-Cause and Cause-Specific Mortality.** *JAMA Internal Medicine,* 2016 DOI: 10.1001/jamainternmed.2016.4182

proteins, like processed and even unprocessed red meats versus plant-based, found trends in plant-based proteins and lower risk of mortality. There is a suggestion to replace some proteins with carbohydrates—which produces some health benefits, like weight management, reduced blood pressure, and other cardiovascular issues. This study stated that consuming more plant-sourced protein will help you have healthier well-being.

Apparently, going plant-based will save trillions of dollars, millions of lives, and very possibly the Earth. A study[8] done at Oxford University compared three scenarios pertaining to veganism: Researchers compared the effects of veganism and global mortality rates, greenhouse gas emissions, and health from an economic standpoint. A world-wide adoption of a plant-based diet predicted to prevent 8.1 million deaths per annum and reduce deaths from all causes by 10% by 2050. Adopting a plant-based diet will reduce food-related greenhouse gases by 70% by 2050.

---

[8] Analysis and valuation of the health and climate change cobenefits of dietary change

Marco Springmann, H. Charles J. Godfray, Mike Rayner, and Peter Scarborough

PNAS April 12, 2016. 113 (15) 4146-4151; published ahead of print March 21, 2016.

https://doi.org/10.1073/pnas.1523119113

Also, going plant-based is projected to save $1067 billion USD a year in costs related to health care. Going plant-based could literally save the world. This study is basically saying that the consumption of animal products causes an obscene amount of health problems.

Chapter Three:

Basic Four-Week Meal Plan

(also, an explanation of some vital vitamins)

(The following meal plan is not designed for weight loss or to build muscle. It is not a low-fat meal plan although you may take out or add any of the ingredients as you see fit. This is not a low-carb meal plan, you can always add more produce. Also, this is not a super-high protein plan meant for pregnant women or athletes. If you are either of these, I suggest adding more protein.)

Breakfast is absolutely the most important meal of the day. You fast for about eight hours while you sleep and when you wake up your blood sugar will be low. Even though you may not be hungry, it is important to get a little something in your stomach for fuel for your body. Your first meal should consist of protein-dense, high-fiber ingredients. These two will help keep you full and energized for the day ahead. Eating five or six small meals throughout the day will give you the boosts you need to not crash hallway through your workload. Drinking lots of water is equally important. Sometimes dehydration will mask itself as hunger.

There are a few nutrients and vitamins that will most likely come up in conversation a lot as a plant-based eater; These include vitamin D, Iron, Protein, and B12.

Vitamin D: Required to be able to absorb calcium properly. Ultimately, the best way to get Vitamin D into your system is through sunlight. Every living thing needs sunlight since it is vital for life to exist. It only takes about five to thirty minutes of sunlight twice a week for us to be able to get all the Vitamin D we need. Many plant-based milks and cereals are fortified with vitamin D. Mushrooms are naturally loaded with vitamin D. The best way to get vitamin D is by going outside and soaking up some sun. A plus side to this is the sun keeps depression at bay.

B-12: When it comes to a plant-based diet, B-12 is hard to come by in food…naturally. It is in soil, and I also produced by the bacteria in your gut, so unless you do not want to wash your produce, the best way to get your B-12 is probably through a daily supplement. Since the oral bioavailability is relatively low, try to find one with a relatively high level of a daily value percentage.

Five sources of B12 include:
1. Most plant-based milks are fortified with B12
2. The same goes for most cereals
3. Plant-based butter spreads
4. Nutritional yeast
5. Nori (seaweed)

Protein: The recommended amount of protein for the average woman is approximately 52 grams per day and for the average man, 63 grams per day. There is protein in almost everything a plant-based eater regularly consumes. Despite the controversy, protein is one of the most easily obtainable of the nutrients. Vegetables, fruits, beans, whole grains, legumes, nuts, and seeds sometimes have just some, and others have quite a bit of protein. The typical American diet has almost too much protein. Unless you are pregnant or athletic, you really do not need as much protein as you would think. Diets high in protein tend to increase chances of osteoporosis and kidney disease.

The top 12 food that contains the highest levels of protein are:
1. Black Beans
2. Tofu
3. Nuts
4. Tempeh
5. Chickpeas
6. Broccoli
7. Quinoa
8. Lentils
9. Potatoes
10. Mushrooms
11. Plant-based milk
12. Plant-based yogurt

Iron: Even though iron is the most common nutrient to be deficient in human. When you are a plant-eater, getting plenty of iron into your system is easier than you would imagine. If you pair it with some form of vitamin C, you will not have any problems with anemia; Vitamin C helps your body absorb iron.

Here are the top ten sources of iron:
1. Tomato Paste
2. White Beans
3. Cooked Soybeans
4. Lentils
5. Dried Apricots
6. Spirulina

7. Spinach
8. Quinoa
9. Blackstrap Molasses
10. Prune Juice

Here is a basic Four-Week Meal Plan with recipes from all different sources. If you are not sure of how to make the recipe, there are many different variations from Minimalist Baker, Forks Over Knives, YouTube, or Eat This Much online. It is relatively simple to follow, and there is no right way to go about this plan.

WEEK 1	Breakfast	Snack	Lunch	Snack	Dinner
Monday	Oatmeal with raspberries blueberries chia seeds cinnamon almonds	Blue-Corn Chips, Black Bean Hummus	Jambalaya with Bell Peppers, Chickpeas	Fresh Fruit	Soup: Potatoes, onions, carrots, veggie broth, bay leaf, olive oil, salt, and pepper
Tuesday	Bananas with plant milk and cinnamon	Fruit, Mixed Nuts	Peanut Butter, Banana and Chia seed sandwich	Apple and Broccoli salad with Olive oil, Lemon juice, Salt, and peppercorn dressing	Rice and Black Bean burrito. Add tomatoes, spinach, salsa, avocado.
Wednesday	Oatmeal	Pretzels, carrots, celery, and peanut butter	Spaghetti with Pasta Sauce of your choice	Pretzels and Orange Juice	Quinoa Stuffed Bell Peppers
Thursday	Coconut yogurt with granola	Chips with Hummus	Whole Wheat bagel with almond butter and Banana	Apple and Broccoli Salad	Black Bean Burgers
Friday	Smoothie: Banana, Spinach, blueberries	Pretzels and Orange	Whole wheat toast with	Mixed nuts and fruit	Rice and Veggie soup

		, Hemp Seeds		cacao and almond butter spread with Berries		
Saturday	Oatmeal	Chia, Banana, Almond Butter Wrap	Jambalaya with chickpeas and steamed veggies	Pretzels and Orange	Spaghetti
Sunday	Yogurt and granola	Hummus and chips	Peanut Butter and Jelly Sandwich with fruit	Fresh fruit and steamed veggies	Burritos with Walnut Meat

WEEK 2	Breakfast	Snack	Lunch	Snack	Dinner
Monday	Oatmeal	Apples and peanut butter	Pad Thai	Fresh fruit	Mixed Veggies with Brown Rice and Soy Sauce
Tuesday	Cinnamon Apple Toast	Strawberries and Chocolate Almond Milk	Tomato Soup with whole wheat garlic toast	Fresh fruit and veggies	Steamed Veggies with brown rice and sweet potato fries
Wednesday	Banana Oatmeal Smoothie	Peanut Butter and Celery	Fully Loaded Salad with Balsamic Dressing	Peanut Butter and carrots	Garlic, White wine pasta with Brussel sprouts
Thursday	Granola and coconut yogurt	Fruit and Mixed nuts	Fully loaded burrito	Chocolate Banana Smoothie	Pad Thai
Friday	Overnight Oats	Strawberries and chocolate almond milk	Couscous with pine nuts and bell peppers	Tomato and hummus on rye bread	Mixed veggies with brown rice and soy sauce
Saturday	Banana Almond Butter Toast	Pretzels and Orange	Pad Thai	Mixed Nuts	Spaghetti with Spiralize

					d Zucchini
Sunday	Overnight Oats	Yogurt and Granola	Peanut Butter and Jelly sandwich	Pretzels and Orange	Burritos

WEEK 3	Breakfast	Snack	Lunch	Snack	Dinner
Monday	Banana Oatmeal Smoothie	Spinach Salad with Carrots	Kale and Avocado Salad	Cantaloupe with granola	White Spaghetti
Tuesday	High Protein Smoothie with Granola	Peanut Butter and Celery	Avocado Pasta Sauce	Spinach and Tomato Salad	Zucchini Peanut Noodles
Wednesday	Overnight Oatmeal	Spinach and Tomato Salad	Apricot Jam and Almond Butter Sandwich	Cabbage and Carrot Juice with Granola	Sea Salt Edamame and Lemon Cous-Cous salad
Thursday	Raspberry Chia Seed Pudding and Oranges	Basic Green smoothie with Red Bell Peppers	Banana, Peanut Butter, and Raisins with Peanut Butter and Celery	Mixed Nuts	White Spaghetti
Friday	Oatmeal and Apples with Granola	Celery and Hummus	Hummus Pocket Sandwich	Sliced Cucumber and Avocado	Fresh Tomato Pasta, Green beans with olive oil
Saturday	Chocolate milk with oatmeal,	Cantaloupe and Red Pepper	Carrot, Hummus, and avocado	Peanut Butter and Celery	Burritos

	raisins, and dates	and Hummus			
Sunday	Blueberry, Almond Butter protein smoothie	Peanut Butter and Celery	Avocado Pasta Sauce	Cucumber and Tomato toss with Granola	Sweet Potato noodles, Cashew Sauce and Brussel Sprouts

WEEK 4	Breakfast	Snack	Lunch	Snack	Dinner
Monday	Oatmeal with raspberries blueberries chia seeds cinnamon almonds	Blue-Corn Chips, Black Bean Hummus	Jambalaya with Bell Peppers, Chickpeas	Fresh Fruit	Soup: Potatoes, onions, carrots, veggie broth, bay leaf, olive oil, salt, and pepper
Tuesday	Bananas with plant milk and cinnamon	Fruit, Mixed Nuts	Peanut Butter, Banana and Chia seed sandwich	Apple and Broccoli salad with Olive oil, Lemon juice, Salt, and peppercorn dressing	Rice and Black Bean burrito. Add tomatoes, spinach, salsa, avocado.
Wednesday	Oatmeal	Pretzels, carrots, celery, and peanut butter	Spaghetti with Pasta Sauce of your choice	Pretzels and Orange Juice	Quinoa Stuffed Bell Peppers
Thursday	Coconut yogurt with granola	Chips with Hummus	Whole Wheat bagel with almond butter and Banana	Apple and Broccoli Salad	Black Bean Burgers

Friday	Smoothie: Banana, Spinach, blueberries, Hemp Seeds	Pretzels and Orange	Whole wheat toast with cacao and almond butter spread with Berries	Mixed nuts and fruit	Rice and Veggie soup
Saturday	Oatmeal	Chia, Banana, Almond Butter Wrap	Jambalaya, chickpeas, steamed veggies	Pretzels and Orange	Spaghetti
Sunday	Yogurt and granola	Hummus and chips	Peanut Butter and Jelly Sandwich with fruit	Fresh fruit and steamed veggies	Burritos with Walnut Meat

www.ingramcontent.com/pod-product-compliance
Lightning Source LLC
LaVergne TN
LVHW010323070526
838199LV00065B/5643